Modern Otology and Neurotology

Series Editor
Kimitaka Kaga
National Institute of Sensory Organs
National Tokyo Medical Center
Tokyo, Japan

This series plays a role as a clinical reference in the rapidly evolving subspecialty of modern otology and neurotology. Written by prominent academic authorities, this series integrates contents from all fields of medicine and covers every aspect of the field, including surgical issues in pediatric audiology, neurotology and neurology, genetic testing, oncological study in auditory and vestibular organs, geriatric audiology and neurotology, and new clinical application of bone conduction hearing etc. Historical developments and unsolved problems of each field will also be described in detail to help readers' understanding. The editors and contributors hope that this book series will contribute to medical residents and experts of otolaryngology and related clinical medicines in the evaluation of patients with otological and neurotological disorders.

More information about this series at http://www.springer.com/series/10581

Kimitaka Kaga

Editor

Cochlear Implantation in Children with Inner Ear Malformation and Cochlear Nerve Deficiency

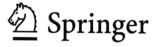 Springer

Editor
Kimitaka Kaga
National Institute of Sensory Organs
National Tokyo Medical Center
Tokyo, Japan

Center for Speech and Hearing Disorders
International University of Health
  and Welfare Clinic
Ohtawara, Japan

Modern Otology and Neurotology
ISBN 978-981-10-9347-0   ISBN 978-981-10-1400-0   (eBook)
DOI 10.1007/978-981-10-1400-0

Printed on acid-free paper

This Springer imprint is published by Springer Nature
The registered company is Springer Nature Singapore Pte Ltd.
The registered company address is: 152 Beach Road, #22-06/08 Gateway East, Singapore 189721,
Singapore

Preface

Cochlear implantation for children with congenital deafness is performed worldwide. The outcome to acquire speech and hearing is epoch-making. Many of those children can learn in mainstream schools. Meanwhile, there are difficult cases of children with complicated inner ear malformation and/or cochlear nerve deficiency. After cochlear implantation, their development of speech and hearing is very slow. Meanwhile, their development of postural control and motor function such as head control and independent walking is also delayed. However, knowledge of basic medicine and data analysis of the outcome of cochlear implant and motor development is insufficient so far.

The purpose of this book is to contribute knowledge of basic and clinical medicine in cochlear implantation and related problems for inner ear malformation and cochlear nerve deficiency.

I thank Ms. Kayoko Sekiguchi for her unlimited contribution in publishing this book.

Tokyo, Japan   Kimitaka Kaga

Contents

Chapter 1
Overview

Kimitaka Kaga

Abstract Classification of inner ear malformation was changed by new study evaluation of the temporal bone morphology since the eighteenth century. Historically, anatomical dissection of temporal bone, X-ray, polytomes, CT, and MRI were clinically used in order. Since introduction of cochlear implant in 1980s, we need more knowledge of inner ear malformation in basic medicine for safer and successful cochlear implantation. Cochlear nerve deficiency was defined as the absence or reduction in caliber of the cochleovestibular nerve (CVN), either more frequency and related to a smaller size of the internal auditory canal. Abnormalities of the CVN are described in 43 % of malformed inner ears, but an absent or hypoplastic nerve can be observed with a cochlear nerve partition. There are urgent problems whether inner ear malformation or cochlear nerve deficiency can be indicated for cochlear implantation and acquired speech and hearing in children as the outcome or not.

Keywords Inner ear malformation • Mondini • Jackler's classification • Sennaroglu's classification • Cochlear nerve deficiency

Before cochlear implantation, inner ear malformation was classified into Michel type, Scheibe type, Mondini type, Alexander type, and others. However, after cochlear implantation, this old classification of inner ear malformation is not insufficient for diagnosis and choice of an electrode of cochlear implant. In 1987, Professor Jackler of Stanford University in the USA reported a new classification to consider cochlear implant [1]. Later in 2002, Professor Sennaroglu of Hacettepe University in Turkey reported more detailed classification of inner ear malformation

K. Kaga, M.D., Ph.D. (✉)
National Institute of Sensory Organs, National Tokyo Medical Center,
2-5-1 Higashigaoka, Meguro-Ku, Tokyo 152-8902, Japan

Center for Speech and Hearing Disorders, International University of Health
and Welfare Clinic, 2600-6 Kitakanemaru, Ohtawara, Tochigi 324-0011, Japan
e-mail: kaga@kankakuki.go.jp

© Springer Science+Business Media Singapore 2017
K. Kaga (ed.), *Cochlear Implantation in Children with Inner Ear Malformation and Cochlear Nerve Deficiency*, Modern Otology and Neurotology,
DOI 10.1007/978-981-10-1400-0_1

and cochlear nerve deficiency for cochlear implant [2]. Since introduction of cochlear implant, it is not rare to encounter various kinds of inner ear malformation and cochlear nerve deficiency. Because of safe and successful cochlear implantation, we need more knowledge of basic medicine of inner ear malformation and cochlear nerve deficiency from views of embryology, surgical skills, and outcome of speech and hearing in each type. These reasons are the background of this book, and the purpose is to inform the updated knowledge.

Cochlear nerve deficiency is diagnosed in deaf children by temporal bone CT or MRI which reveals decrease in number of cochlear or vestibular nerve. It is difficult to predict outcomes of cochlear implant because it depends on number of cochlear nerve. Meantime, acquisition of head control and independent walking are marked by delayed time because of vestibular nerve deficiency. Besides auditory evaluation, vestibular function study is important because of semicircular canal malformation or vestibular nerve deficiency complicates frequently and head control and independent walking are delayed to acquire. Then, we emphasize that evaluation of vestibular function is very important as well as evaluation of auditory function in children with inner ear malformation and cochlear nerve deficiency. This overview describes the history of inner ear malformation and cochlear nerve deficiency in otology.

1.1   Inner Ear Malformation

1.1.1   The Eighteenth Century: "Dissection of the Temporal Bone by Mondini (Figs. 1.1 and 1.2)"

Who was the first to describe the inner ear anomaly in the medical history? That is C. Mondini (1729–1803) in Italy. Professor H. Edamatsu of Toho University of Medicine in Tokyo investigated and reported Mondini's article in Latin [3].

In 1791, Mondini wrote the Latin article entitled *Anatomica Surdi Nati Sectio* [4]. It became the first report of the dissection of the temporal bone in an 8 year-old boy with congenital deafness and reported the anatomical findings of the inner ear anomaly. Mondini's original paper is a historical one for ontological researchers, but it has been difficult, indeed rather impossible, to read for a long time. We fortunately had the chance to review the original copy of the paper.

The summary of Mondini's report described several conditions: there was a large opening of the vestibular aqueduct, labyrinth fluid was escaping from the enlarged vestibular aqueduct, and the cochlea consisted of only one and a half turns, among others. According to his paper, the common cavity is not an inner ear anomaly of the Mondini type. Currently, recent progress in three-dimensional imaging can detect and visualize the fine and detailed structure of the inner ear. Therefore, imaging diagnosis is able to discriminate Mondini anomalies from other types.

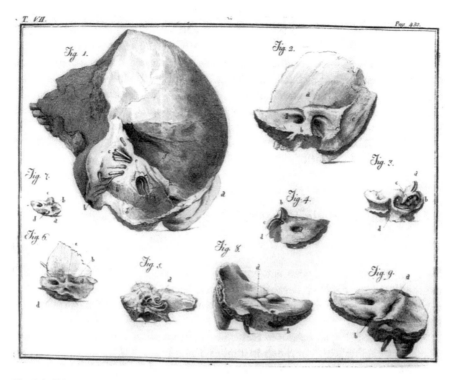

Fig. 1.1 Dissection of temporal bone by Mondini

a

b

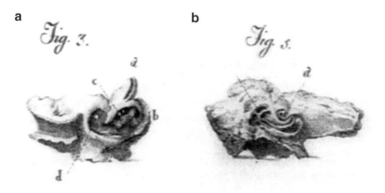

Fig. 1.2 Illustration of the cochlea by Mondini

In 1904, Alexander described incomplete development of the bony and membranous labyrinth with basal turn only and interscalar septum in the upper turns resulting gross distention of the endolymphatic sac [5].

In modern age, Mondini's anomaly of the inner ear is variously modified and misinterpreted. However, we should return the Mondini's original article.

1.1.2   The Nineteenth Century: "Temporal Bone Histology"

In 1863, Michel reported complete lack of development of the inner ear [6]. Later, in 1964, Jorgensen et al. [7] and, in 1971, Black et al. [8] described agenesis of the labyrinth in temporal bone pathology.

In 1892, Scheibe described the malformation limited to the cochlea and saccule with membranous cochlea-saccular aplasia and normal bony labyrinth [9].

In 1965, Shuknecht et al. suggested the concept of cochlea-saccular degeneration in congenital deafness [10].

1.1.3   The Twentieth Century: "X-ray and CT of Temporal Bone"

X-ray polytome and CT scan and MRI developed new classification of inner ear malformation and cochlear nerve deficiency. Development of cochlear implants has needed precise anatomical structure of cochlea for insertion of electrodes into cochlear turns.

In 1987, Jackler et al. proposed congenital malformation of the inner ear: a classification based on embryogenesis in Table 1.1 and Fig. 1.3 [1]. This classification was proposed by polytomes or CT scans considering embryogenesis of cochlea and vestibular end organs.

Table 1.1 Classification of congenital malformation of the inner ear [1]

A. With an absent or malformed cochlea
1. Complete labyrinthine aplasia (Michel deformity): no inner ear development
2. Cochlear aplasia: no cochlea, normal or malformed vestibule and semicircular canals
3. Cochlear hypoplasia: small cochlear bud, normal or malformed vestibule, and semicircular canals
4. Incomplete partition: small cochlea with incomplete or no interscalar septum, normal or malformed vestibule, and semicircular canals
5. Common cavity; cochlea and vestibule form a common cavity without internal architecture; normal or malformed semicircular canals
B. With a normal cochlea
1. Vestibule-lateral semicircular canal dysplasia; enlarged vestibule with a short, dilated lateral semicircular canal; remaining semicircular canals are normal
2. Enlarged vestibular aqueduct; accompanied by normal semicircular canals, normal or enlarged vestibule

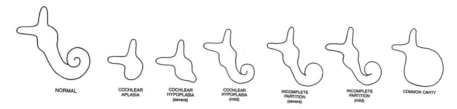

Fig. 1.3 Cochlear malformations; these drawings represent a composite of sequential slices derived from an anteroposterior polytomographic examination [1]

1.1.4 The Twenty-First Century: "High-Resolution CT and MRI of the Temporal Bone"

Multichannel cochlear implants have been introduced in order to recover hearing in deaf children and adults in the world since 1980. This hearing technology is epoch-making in hearing science. Indication of cochlear implant has been extended to more difficult cases with inner ear malformation or cochlear nerve deficiency.

In 2002, Sennaroglu and Saatci proposed a new classification of cochleovestibular malformation. This new classification is based on embryogenesis of labyrinth, vestibular end organs, cochleovestibular nerve, and inner auditory canal and images of CT scans. Before decision of cochlear implantation, this classification is worldwidely used (Figs. 1.4 and 1.5) [2].

1.2 Cochlear Nerve Deficiency (CND)

Vincenti et al. recognized [11] that Shelton et al. [12] first suggested cochlear nerve absence as an explanation for the lack of auditory response to electric stimulation in three children with narrow inner auditory canal (IAC) who underwent cochlear implantation. Since then, several reports on cochlear implantation in CND have been published with generally poor results.

Glastonbury et al. [13] defined cochlear nerve "deficiency" as the absence or the reduction in caliber of the cochleovestibular nerve (CVN), either congenital (more frequent and related to a smaller size of the IAC) or acquired. They also described the so-called isolated cochlea, in which the medial opening of the modiolar canal is absent.

Abnormalities of the CVN are described in 43 % of malformed inner ears [14], but an absent or hypoplastic nerve can be observed also with a normal cochlear partition [15] because the embryologic development of the cochlea is independent of its innervation [16].

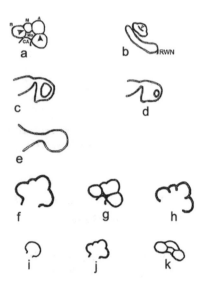

Fig. 1.4 Schematic representation of the normal cochlea and cochlea malformations [2]. (**a**) Normal cochlea, midmodiolar section *MO* modiolus, *CA* cochlear aperture, *B* basal turn, *M* middle turn, *A* apical turn, *arrowheads* = interscalar septa. (**b**) Normal cochlea, inferior section passing through the round window niche (RWN). *Arrowhead* interscalar septum between middle and apical turns. (**c**) Cochlear aplasia with normal vestibule. (**d**) Cochlear aplasia with enlarged vestibule. (**e**) Common cavity. (**f**) Incomplete partition type I (IP-I). (**g**) Incomplete partition type II (IP-II). (**h**) Incomplete partition type III (IP-III). (**i**) Cochlear hypoplasia, bud type (type I). (**j**) Cochlear hypoplasia, cystic cochlea type (type II) (hypoplasia (type II)). (**k**) Cochlear hypoplasia, with less than 2 turns (type III) (hypoplasia (type III))

Fig. 1.5 Defect at the lateral end of the internal auditory canal. Incomplete partition type I (**a**) and common cavity (**b**) (*C* cochlea, **defect*, *CC* common cavity) [2]

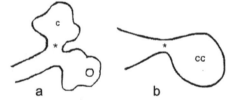

Zanetli et al. [17] consider that the classification of CVN dysplasia was proposed first by Govaerts et al. [18]. This useful and practical classification has three categories based on the MRI findings:

- *Type I*: total absence of the CVN
- *Type IIa*: cochlear nerve branch absent or hypoplastic, vestibular nerve present, and dysplasia of the cochleovestibular labyrinth
- *Type IIb*: cochlear nerve branch absent or hypoplastic, vestibular nerve present, and normal morphology of the cochleovestibular labyrinth

Colletti et al. [19] reported that the possibility of finding of a person with a malformed or even normal cochlea, agenesia of the cochlear nerve, and normal cochlear nuclei is not a biologic absurdity. In fact, comparative anatomic and embryologic studies have shown that the cochlea develops independently of the nerve, and the nerve has no trophic effects on the nuclei [20].

From a view of development of inner ear and auditory nerve, Colletti et al. [19] illustrated that the cochlea begins to develop at the third embryonic week with the appearance of the otic placode, which transforms into the otic vesicle that gives rise to the sacculus, utriculus, semicircular canals, cochlea, and endolymphatic duct. When the cochlea is fully developed, the neural epithelium starts to appear at the ninth week. Neuroblasts of the cochlear ganglion are separated from the otic epithelium and give rise to fibers that grow centrally into the brainstem and peripherally back into otic epithelium. It was once believed that the development of a normal cochlea depended on neural innervation. Embryologic studies on explanted chicken otic vesicles demonstrated that the inner ear development and the differentiation of the hair cells are locally controlled and do not depend on any neuronal stimulus or trigger or trophic effect. Conversely, the otic vesicle and the developing cochlea release a growth factor that is essential for the cytodifferentiation and survival of the afferent neurons.

These embryologic features may explain both the findings in patients with an abnormal cochlea or absence of the cochlea and absence of the cochlear nerve and the findings in patients with a normal cochlea and absence of the cochlear nerve caused by a disturbance in the production or release of this nerve growth factor.

Outcomes of speech and hearing in patients with cochlear nerve deficiency after cochlear implants are various. Zanetti et al. [17] reported achieving satisfactory results by cochlear implantation in type IIb dysplasia of the cochleovestibular nerves even when the imaging of CVN is doubtful and electrophysiological tests are disproportionate.

Vincenti et al. [11] reported on auditory performance after cochlear implantation in children with cochlear nerve deficiency. The outcomes are extremely variable, but all patients in their eases device benefit in everyday life. In their opinion, cochlear implantation can be an available option in children with cochlear nerve deficiency, but careful counseling to the family on possible restricted benefit is needed.

Finally, it is recommended the illustration of the fundus of the internal auditory canal by Soudant is very useful anatomically to understand various types of cochlear nerve deficiency [21] (Fig. 1.6).

Fig. 1.6 Illustration of the
fundus of internal auditory
canal [21]. *1* VII, facial
nerve; *2* facial nerve; *3*
VIII, cochlear nerve; *4*
VIII, vestibular nerve

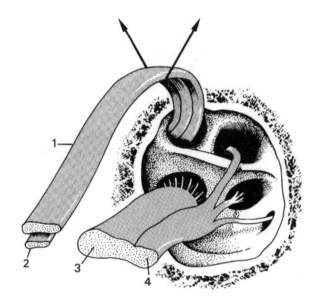

References

1. Jackler RE, Luxford WM, House WF. Congenital malformations of the inner ear, a classification based on embryogenesis. Laryngoscope. 1987;97 Suppl 4:2–14. doi:10.1002/lary.5540971301.
2. Sennaroglu L, Saatci IA. New classification of cochleovestibular malformations. Laryngoscope. 2002;112:2230–41. doi:10.1097/00005537-200212000-00019.
3. Edamatsu H, Yasuda M, Sasaki Y, Kobayashi M, Seto Y, Suetsugu T, et al. The original paper on the Mondini's anomaly of the inner ear and three dimensional imaging. Otolaryngologica Pract Suppl. 2015;143:24–8.
4. Mondini C. Academia surdi nadti sectio. De bononiensi scientarium et atrium, vol. 7. Bologna: instituto atque academia commentarii; 1791. p. 419–31.
5. Alexander GT. Zur pathologie und pathologischen anatomie der kongenitalen taubheit. Arch Ohren Nasen Kehlkogfheilkd. 1904;61:183–291.
6. Michel EM. Gas med Strasbourg. (Abstract: Arch F Ohrenhelk 1: 353–354) 1864;3: 55–58, 1863.
7. Jorgensen MB, Kristensen HK, Buch NH. Thaldomide-induced aplasia of the inner ear. J Laryngol Otol. 1964;78:1095–101. http://dx.doi.org/10.1017/S0022215100063234.
8. Black FO, Bergstrom LV, Downs M, Hemmenway W. Congenital deafness-a new approach. Boulder: Colorado University Press; 1971.
9. Scheibe A. Ein fall von taubstnmmheit mit acusticusatirophie und bildungsanomailien in haustigen labyrinth beiderseits. Z Hals Nasen Ohrenheilkd. 1892;22:11–23.
10. Shuknecht HF, Igarasi M, Chasin WD. Inner ear malformation in leukemia. A case report. Laryngoscope. 1965;75:662–8. doi:10.1288/00005537-196504000-00007.c.
11. Vincenti V, Ormitti F, Ventura E, Guida M, Piccinini A, Pasanisi E. Cochlear implantation in children with cochlear nerve deficiency. Int J Pediatr Otorhinolaryngol. 2014;78:912–7. doi:10.1016/j.ijporl.2014.03.003.

12. Shelton C, Luxford WM, Tonokawa LL, et al. The narrow internal auditory canal in children: A contraindication to cochlear implants. Otolarygol Head Neck Surg. 1989;100:227–31. doi:10.1177/019459988910000310.
13. Glastonbury CM, Davidson HC, Harnsberger HR, Butler J, Kertesz TR, Shelton C. Imaging findings of cochlear nerve deficiency. Am J Neuroradiol. 2002;23:635–43.
14. Westerhof JP, Rademaker J, Weber WP, Becker H. Congenital malformations of the inner ear and the vestibulocochlear nerve in children with sensorineural hearing loss: evaluation with CT and MRI. J Comput Assist Tomogr. 2001;25:719–26.
15. Casselman JW, Offeciers FE, Govaerts PJ, Kuhweide R, Geldof H, Somers T, et al. Aplasia and hypoplasia of the vestibulocochlear nerve: diagnosis with MR imaging. Radiology. 1997;202:773–81. doi:10.1148/radiology.202.3.9051033.
16. Lefebvre PP, Leprince P, Weber T, Rigo JM, Dleree P, Moonen G. Neuronotrophic effect of developing otic vesicle on cochlea-vestibular neurons: evidence for nerve growth factor involvement. Brain Res. 1990;507:254–60. doi:10.1016/0006-8993(90)90279-K.
17. Zanetti D, Guida M, Barezzani MG, Campovecchi C, Nassif N, Pinelli L, Giordano L, Olioso G. Favorable outcome of cochlear implant in VIIIth nerve deficiency. Otol Neurotol. 2006;27:815–23. doi:10.1097/01.mao.0000227899.80656.1d.
18. Govaerts PJ, Casselman J, Daemers K, De Beukelaer C, Yperman M, De Ceulaer G. Cochlear implants in aplasia and hypoplasia of the cochleovestibular nerve. Otol Neurotol. 2003;24:887–91.
19. Colletti VC, Carner M, Fiorino F, Sacchetto L, Miorelli V, Orsi A, et al. Hearing restoration with auditory brainstem implant in three children with cochlear nerve deficiency. Otol Neurotol. 2002;23:682–93.
20. Van De Water TR. Effects of removal of the statoacoustic ganglion complex upon the growing otocyst. Ann Otol Rhinol Laryngol. 1976;85(6 Suppl 33 Pt 2):2–31.
21. Soudant J. Chirurgie du nerf facial. Arnet Paris, 1990, pp 4.

Chapter 2
Embryology of Inner Ear and Its Malformation

Kimitaka Kaga

Abstract Embryologically, the cochlea and the auditory sensory cells develop until 24 weeks and are completed at relatively late stage of the fetus compared with the vestibular organs and vestibular sensory cells.

Neuronal myelination in human brain starts around gestation month 4. The auditory system belongs to older strains in the order of phylogenesis, and both neuronal myelination and development start late. The role of the auditory sense in the cochlea is classified into auditory perception and directional hearing in newborns and infants. In development of the brain, hearing can accelerate speech, language, sound localization, and selective attention.

Keywords Cochlear • Hearing • Inner ear malformation • Auditory system • Sound localization • Vestibular system

2.1 Anatomical Development of the Cochlea and Auditory System

The timetable of major events in development of the human inner ear can give us various clues to understand inner ear malformation and cochlear nerve deficiency (Table 2.1) [1]. Meanwhile, the relationship between maturation of the central auditory system and the development has been explained by Flechsig in 1920 [2]. Later, Yakovlev et al. illustrated progression of myelination of the various nervous systems and the age of its start and completion including the statoacoustic system in 1967 [3].

K. Kaga (✉)
National Institute of Sensory Organs, National Tokyo Medical Center,
2-5-1 Higashigaoka, Meguro-Ku, Tokyo 152-8902, Japan

Center for Speech and Hearing Disorders, International University of Health and Welfare Clinic, 2600-6 Kitakanemaru, Ohtawara, Tochigi 324-0011, Japan
e-mail: kaga@kankakuki.go.jp

© Springer Science+Business Media Singapore 2017
K. Kaga (ed.), *Cochlear Implantation in Children with Inner Ear Malformation and Cochlear Nerve Deficiency*, Modern Otology and Neurotology,
DOI 10.1007/978-981-10-1400-0_2

11

Table. 2.1 Timetable of major events in the human inner ear development [1]

Fetal week	Inner ear
3rd	Auditory placode; auditory pit
4th	Auditory vesicle (otocyst); vestibular-cochlear division
6th	Utricle and saccule present; semicircular canal begins
7th	One cochlear coil present; sensory cells in utricle and saccule
8th	Ductus reuniens present; sensory cells in semicircular canals
11th	Two and one-half cochlear coils present; sensory cells in semicircular canals
12th	Sensory cells in the cochlea; membranous labyrinth complete; otic capsule begins to ossify
20th	Maturation of the internal ear; internal ear adult size

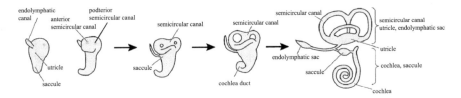

Fig. 2.1 The development of the human labyrinth

2.1.1 Development of the Cochlea and Myelination of the Auditory System

Embryologically the cochlea and their sensory cells develop and are completed at a relatively late stage of fetus compared with the vestibular organ (Fig. 2.1) [4]. The otocyst separates from the neural crest around gestation week 4, and the endolymphatic duct develops around gestation week 5. The membranous labyrinth develops into nearly the shape and size of the adult around gestation week 12, and the Corti's organ is already complete at approximately gestation week 24 (Fig. 2.2). The whole size of the cochlea completes early at week 24 and does not change later (Fig. 2.3). In other words, the cochlea of a newborn has been morphologically completed by this time [1, 5]. This developmental plan in the cochlea suggests that inner ear malformation can be caused by arrest of process of cochlear development at very early gestation. Therefore, the reasons why there are many kinds of inner ear malformations must be caused by different times of arrest of fetus development.

Scarpa's ganglion is located in the modiolus inside the cochlea. This ganglion markedly increases its size with progression of gestation. Its size at week 39 is fourfold of that at week 13 [5].

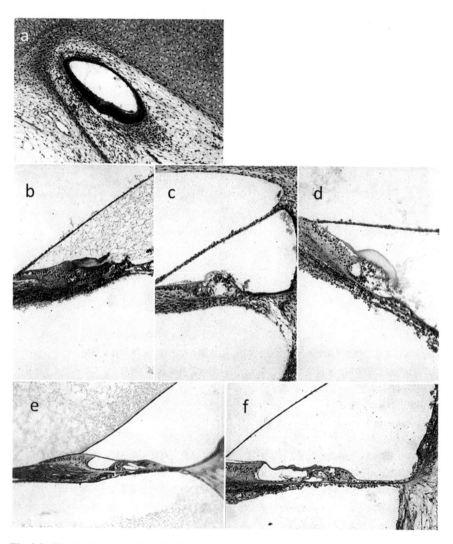

Fig. 2.2 The development of the Corti's organ. It is complete at approximately gestation week 24. (**a**) week 13, (**b**) week 17, (**c**) week 19, (**d**) week 21, (**e**) week 24, (**f**) newborn

2.1.2 Inner Ear Malformation and Arrest of Development of the Inner Ear

Jackler et al. presented a hypothesis of inner ear malformation from a view of development of inner ear in embryogenesis [6]: At the third gestational week, a failure of development would result in complete labyrinthine aplasia of the Michel type (Fig. 2.4).

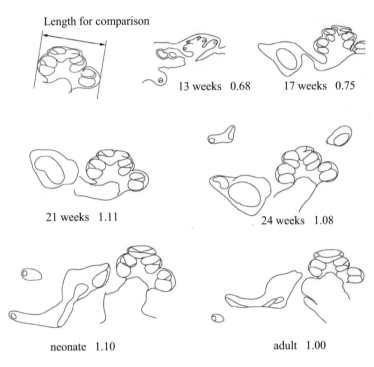

Length for comparison

13 weeks 0.68   17 weeks 0.75

21 weeks 1.11   24 weeks 1.08

neonate 1.10   adult 1.00

Fig. 2.3 Size changes of the cochlea in development of gestational weeks. Adult size is measured as 1.0 [13]

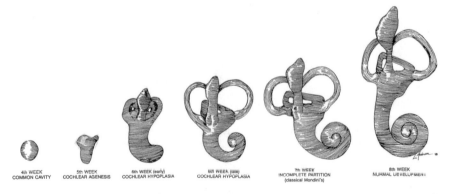

Fig. 2.4 Embryogenesis of cochlear malformation by Jackler et al. [6]

A lack of normal differentiation beyond the fourth-week stage may result in the persistence of a large cloaca as seen in the common cavity cases: arrested development of the cochlear bud at this stage also would result in cochlear aplasia with preservation of the semicircular canals and vestibule.

A cessation of cochlear development during the sixth week may represent the various degrees of cochlear hypoplasia.

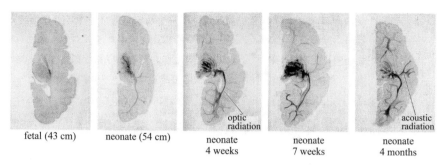

fetal (43 cm)   neonate (54 cm)   neonate   neonate   neonate
                                                4 weeks   7 weeks   4 months

Fig. 2.5 Flechsig's study on developmental brain and myelination [2]

At the seventh week stage, an arrest of maturation may result in the classical Mondini's deformity as a small cochlea with an incomplete intracochlear partition.

Other malformations may result from aberrant rather than arrested development or a combination of the two. This may account for unusual anomalies, such as extra-cochlear turns, cochlear duplication, and other such rarities.

In the sixth gestational week, the semicircular canals begin as folded evaginations of membrane from the vestibular appendage. Failure of these epithelial folds to form would result in complete absence of the involved semicircular canal (SCC). The superior SCC is the first to form, followed by the posterior (PCC) and then lateral canal (LCC).

It is interesting to note that many patients had inner ear abnormalities, involving combinations of the cochlea, semicircular canals, and vestibular aqueduct perhaps due to a common developmental precursor or to a shared susceptibility to some teratogenic agent.

2.1.3 Development of the Central Auditory Pathway

Myelination in human brain starts around gestation month 4, but full-fledged development starts after birth and continues through infancy into puberty. However, myelination does not progress at the same time, and myelination is completed early or later depending on the strain, following a certain order. The rule applies here, in principle, that developmentally older strains are completed sooner also in individual development. Flechsig [2] concluded that the fascicle becomes completely functional after completion of myelination (Fig. 2.5). In fact, function and myelination are closely related, and myelination tends to be completed sooner in strains with an earlier start of function.

The central auditory pathway belongs to new strains in the order of phylogenesis, and both myelination and development start late [7].

The myelination of the auditory system starts after that of the visual system and completes around 1 year after birth.

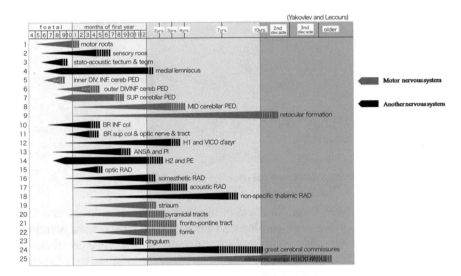

Fig. 2.6 The myelination cycle [3]. The width and length of graphs show the progression of stainability of myelinated nerve fibers and the intensity of concentration. *Dark shaded* portions at the far right indicate the age when myelination has been completed, by comparing specimens of fetuses, newborns, and adults

Yakovlev et al. [3] reported in their study of myelination that the duration required for completion of the myelin sheath differs, as each fiber bundle starts developing a myelin sheath at a different time. Each fiber bundle follows a predetermined cycle of myelination, which is called the "myelogenetic cycle" (Fig. 2.6). For instance, myelination of motor nerves has a short cycle (between gestation month 5 and 10), whereas myelination of the sensory nerves starts later and takes longer to complete (between gestation month 6 and 4 years of age). Myelination of the stato-acoustic tectum and tegmentum is short-cycled and occurs between gestation month 6 and 9.

In other words, myelination of the brainstem auditory pathway starts during the prenatal period and is completed by birth. On the other hand, myelination of acoustic radiation in the cerebral hemisphere starts after birth and is completed by 3 years of age. On the other hand, the duration of the cycle of brainstem reticular formation is longer (1 month to 10 years of age), and that of association area is completed at 20 years of age.

2.1.4 As Developmental Arrest of the Inner Ear, Common Cavity, and Cochlear Nerve Deficiency May Occur

Among inner ear malformations, common cavity is one of the most severe abnormalities.

Common cavity deformity has been reported to occur in 2 % of patients with congenital profound sensorineural hearing loss [8]. In this inner ear malformation, the cochlea and vestibules form a common cavity, usually lacking an internal architecture. This deformity is regarded as hypoplasia of the cochleovestibular nerve or complete aplasia of the cochleovestibular nerve [9]. In embryos of approximately 5 weeks or less, the saccule is demarcated from the remainder of the vesicle: it sends out a single ventral evagination, the primordium of the cochlear duct. Common cavity deformity most probably results from an arrest in otocyst development during the fourth gestational week.

In the human early development stage, neuroblasts of the cochlear ganglion separate from the otic epithelium at approximately the fourth gestational week. The cochleovestibular nerve (CVN) develops at approximately 9 weeks of gestation [10]. Sennaroglu et al. reported that a patient with a common cavity, who had a "common CVN" without branching into the cochlear and vestibular nerves, showed good benefit from cochlear implantation, but showed nystagmus after cochlear implantation [11]. This suggests that the cochlear and vestibular nerve fibers must be present in their cochlear nerve deficiency. However, the function of the inferior vestibular nerve remains unknown.

2.1.5 Conduction Speed of Nerve Impulse Before and After Myelination

Finally, it is important to know conductive speed of nerve impulse before and after completion of myelination. Before myelination, nerve impulse is conducted through axon, and the conductive speed of nerve impulse is 3–5 km/h. After completion of myelination, the conductive speed of nerve impulse is 50–400 km/h. This difference suggests how myelination is important to study brain neuronal network and appearance of each brain function including speech, language, learning, memory, thinking, and others [12].

References

1. Northern JL, Downs MP. Hearing in children. Baltimore: Lippincott William & Wilkins; 1974.
2. Flechsig P. Anatomie des menschen Gehirns und Rückenmarks auf Myelogenetischer Grundlage. Leipzig: Georg Thime; 1920.
3. Yakovlev PI, Lecotus A-R. The myelogenetic cycles of regional maturation of the brain. In: Minkovoski A, editor. Regional development of the brain in early life. Oxford: Blackwell Scientific Publicaitons; 1967.
4. Nomura Y, Hiraide F, Harada T. New atlas of otology. Tokyo: Springer; 1992.
5. Kaga K, Sakurai H, Ogawa Y, Mizutani T, Toriyama M. Morphological changers of vestibular ganglion cells in human fetuses and in pediatric patients. Int J Pediatr Otorhinolaryngol. 2001;60:11–20. doi:10.1016/S0165-5876(01)00493-1.

6. Jackler RE, Luxford WM, House WF. Congenital malformations of the inner ear, a classification based on embryogenesis. Laryngoscope. 1987;97 Suppl 4:2–14. doi:10.1002/lary.5540971301.
7. Kamoshita S. Development of neurological system. Progression of pediatric neurology. Volume 1, Diagnosis and treatment. Tokyo, 1972.
8. Buchman CA, Copeland BK, Yu KK, Brown CJ, Carrasco VN, Pillsbury III HC. Cochlear implantation in children with congenital inner ear malformations. Laryngoscope. 2004;114:309–16. doi:10.1097/00005537-200402000-00025.
9. Manolidis S, Tonini R, Spitzer J. Endoscopically guided placement of prefabricated cochlear implant electrodes in a common cavity malformation. Int J Pediatr Otorhinolaryngol. 2006;70:595–6. doi:http://dx.doi.org/10.1016/j.ijporl.2005.07.004.
10. Papsin BC. Cochlear implantation in children with anomalous cochleovestibular anatomy. Laryngoscope. 2006;115:1–26. doi:10.1097/00005537-200501001-00001.
11. Sennaroglu L, Gursel B, Sennaroglu G, Yucel E, Saatci I. Vestibular stimulation after cochlear implantation in common cavity deformity. Otolaryngol Head Neck Surg. 2001;125:408–10. doi:10.1067/mhn.2001.118072.
12. Tanji jin. Five years of integrated brain study. Grant-in-aid for scientific on priority areas. The 5th area. Research Bulletin, p. 1–32.
13. Sasaki T, Kaga K. Hearing of the newborn-the basis of form and function. ENTONI. 2004;33:1–8.

Chapter 3
Embryology of Cochlear Nerve and Its Deficiency

Irumee Pai

Abstract Most studies on development of the human auditory system and hearing loss have to date focused on the sensory apparatus, the cochlea. With advancements in magnetic resonance imaging (MRI), there has recently been increasing interest in the subject of cochlear nerve deficiency (CND) and dysfunction. Cochlear nerve deficiency (CND) amongst individuals with congenital sensorineural hearing loss (SNHL) is not as rare as previously thought, with prevalence as high as 18–21 % reported amongst cochlear implant recipients. Cochlear nerve (CN) morphogenesis is a complex process involving cell populations from two disparate progenitors of the otic placode and neural crest cells. In the first trimester, the basic foundation of the auditory pathway is laid down, with the vestibulocochlear ganglion cells delaminating from the otocyst and establishing peripheral and central connections with the developing cochlea and brainstem, respectively. The second trimester is a period of proliferation, growth and myelination. As the number of axons is pruned back closer to the adult level, myelination begins in the intra-cochlear portion of CN and extends proximally. In the third trimester, further maturation of the neuronal connections in conjunction with paralleled development of the cochlea and brainstem leads to emergence of foetal responses to auditory stimuli. Based on the currently available knowledge of the embryological development of CN, various phenotypes of CND are discussed. It is hoped that better understanding of CN ontogenesis will not only lead to further refinement of auditory implant candidacy but also open doors to potential regeneration therapies such as stem cell therapy in the future.

Keywords Embryology • Development • Cochlear • Nerve • Deficiency

I. Pai (✉)
St. Thomas' Hospital, Westminster Bridge Road, London SE1 7EH, UK
e-mail: Irumee.Pai@gstt.nhs.uk

© Springer Science+Business Media Singapore 2017
K. Kaga (ed.), *Cochlear Implantation in Children with Inner Ear Malformation and Cochlear Nerve Deficiency*, Modern Otology and Neurotology,
DOI 10.1007/978-981-10-1400-0_3

19

3.1 Introduction

Hearing loss is the commonest congenital sensory deficit, affecting approximately 1 in 1000 live births in most developed countries. In certain communities, the incidence may be up to three to four times higher. In the majority of cases of congenital sensorineural hearing loss (SNHL), the location of malfunction is within the inner ear. It is therefore not surprising that most studies on development of the human auditory system have to date focused on the sensory apparatus, the cochlea.

More recently, there has been increasing interest in the subject of cochlear nerve deficiency and dysfunction. Advancements in magnetic resonance imaging (MRI) techniques mean that it is now possible to clearly visualise the cochlear nerve (CN) separate from the facial nerve and the superior and inferior branches of the vestibular nerve within the lateral portion of the internal auditory meatus. As access to MRI continues to improve around the world, it has become the imaging modality of choice in many centres for aetiological investigation of SNHL and as part of cochlear implant assessment. As a result, abnormalities of the cochlear nerve are coming under increasing attention, although their clinical implications are not always clear. Cochlear nerve deficiency (CND) amongst individuals with congenital SNHL is not as rare as previously thought, with prevalence as high as 18–21 % reported amongst cochlear implant recipients in recent studies [1–3]. Furthermore, as outcomes of cochlear implantation improve overall and implant candidacy continues to expand, there is closer scrutiny of potential prognostic factors, including congenital anomalies of CN as well as those of the inner ear, which may negatively impact on the implant outcome. Such is particularly the case when there is a significant doubt as to the presence of a functional connection between the cochlea and the brainstem, and an auditory brain stem implant may need to be considered as a potentially better option.

This chapter provides an overview of the current knowledge of the embryological development of CN and discusses its clinical relevance.

3.2 Embryology

The vestibulocochlear nerve (VCN), like all peripheral nerves, consists of neurons and supporting glial cells [4]. Peripheral glial cells include Schwann cells, which surround and myelinate neuronal axons and neurites, and satellite cells, which support ganglionic neuronal cell bodies. The glial cell component of VCN arises from neural crest cell (NCC) progenitors of the embryonic ectoderm [5–7]. It is commonly held that the neurons of VCN originate almost exclusively from the otic placode [7–10]. However, it has recently been suggested that a significant proportion of VCN neurons may be traced back to NCC or another type of migratory neuroepithelial cells [11]. Throughout all stages of VCN morphogenesis, there is extensive interaction between the two cell populations from the otic placode and NCC progenitors, developing very much in tandem [12].

3.2.1 First Trimester

In the human embryo, the otic placode begins to develop around 3 weeks of gestation (WG) as a thickening of the epidermis on either side of the head. It soon invaginates and separates from the surface ectoderm to form a spherical epithelial structure, referred to as the otic vesicle or otocyst [13–15]. By 4 WG, a group of cells have delaminated from the otocyst and become stationed between the developing inner ear and hindbrain. After undergoing cell proliferation and differentiation, these neuroblasts give rise to the vestibulocochlear ganglion [16–18].

The ganglion cells that will develop into the cochlear division of the nerve project back to the developing cochlea and wind around the modiolus, forming the spiral ganglia. The immature neurons begin to establish polarity by extending their processes in two directions, peripherally towards the inner ear and centrally towards the brainstem [18, 19]. The central processes, the axons, are the first to reach their destination, arriving in the brainstem by the fifth to sixth week of foetal development. Within the brainstem, all of the auditory centres and pathways are identifiable by 7–8 WG, with clusters of neurons recognisable as the cochlear nuclei [16]. The dendritic processes directed peripherally penetrate the undifferentiated, primordial organ of Corti at 9 WG. By 10–12 WG, they form rounded synaptic terminals, making contact with the bases of the developing hair cells [18, 20]. It has been shown that the migration, growth and survival of the vestibulocochlear ganglion cells are likely to be dependent on a number of neurotrophic factors, in particular brain-derived neurotrophic factor and neurotrophin-3, expressed by the otocyst [21–23].

Another event of significant clinical relevance around this stage in development is the change in the mesenchyme in association with the early sensory apparatus and neural connections. At 9 WG, the mesenchyme surrounding the otocyst begins to form a cartilaginous matrix, which eventually ossifies and turns into the otic capsule. This chondrogenesis occurs in synchrony with the development of VCN, whose presence inhibits cartilage formation at the medial aspect of the otocyst, eventually leading to the formation of the internal auditory canal (IAC). As with the early development of the vestibulocochlear ganglion cells, which requires various neurotrophic factors produced by the otocyst, the induction of chondrogenesis involves close and reciprocal epithelial-mesenchymal tissue interactions between the otocyst and periotic mesenchyme [24]. The formation of IAC is completed by 5 months of gestational age, and it has been hypothesised that the calibre of the IAC is related to the volume of the migrating VCN fibres [25].

3.2.2 Second Trimester

CN undergoes rapid proliferation and maturation during the second trimester. Around 14 WG, the dendrites extending from the spiral ganglia begin to form synaptic contacts with the inner and outer hair cells of the cochlea. This process of synaptogenesis has been shown to progress along a base-to-apex gradient [26].

The mechanisms by which CN ganglion cells differentiate into type I and type II ganglion cells, establish their connections with the correct, corresponding hair cell types and match the tonotopic development of the cochlea are poorly understood.

During this period, CN not only grows in its diameter, increasing almost three-fold in cross-sectional area between 22 and 28 WG, but also begins to develop a distinct fascicular arrangement of axons surrounded by increasingly compact connective tissue. Ray et al. observed in their study of the development of the human foetal nerve that the number of axons continued to increase until 20 WG and subsequently reduced to the adult level at 22 WG [27].

One of the most significant events during the mid-gestation period is myelination, which is crucial for rapid synchronised conduction. Developing Schwann cells are detected in foetal embryos as early as 12 WG. At 15 WG, clusters of Schwann cells are seen along the axons in the spiral lamina and modiolus, and by 20–22 WG, myelination has begun within the spiral lamina fibres, with a well-defined, close association between the axons and Schwann cells [26–28]. By the 24th week of foetal development, myelin sheaths can be seen to extend along the nerve up to the glial junction at the point where the nerve exits from the temporal bone. The proximal segment of CN beyond this point is supported by oligodendrocytes, but myelination does not begin until later [28]. One of the interesting findings in the study of human foetal CN by Ray et el. was the maturational asymmetry between the left and right sides, with myelination of the right cochlear nerve consistently lagging behind the left until 38 WG [27]. The clinical implications of this observation have yet to be elucidated.

3.2.3   Third Trimester

As both the cochlear nerve and the central neural connections continue to mature functionally as well as structurally, foetal responses to auditory stimuli start to emerge. Using vibroacoustic stimulation during ultrasound imaging, blink-startle responses could be observed in some foetuses as early as 24–25 WG, and the responses were present consistently after 28 WG [29, 30]. Studies in preterm infants show that auditory brainstem responses (ABRs) can be elicited from around 26 weeks of conceptional age and become more consistent from 29 weeks, although they require stronger intensity stimuli at slower rates. The ABR thresholds appear to stabilise approximately at adult values around 35 WG, and the latencies of the various potential components continue to decrease to term [31–33].

3.2.4   Summary

The foundation of CN morphogenesis is laid down in the first trimester, with the otocyst giving rise to and sustaining the vestibulocochlear ganglion cells which migrate and form connections with the early cochlea and brainstem. The second trimester is a period of proliferation and maturation. Synaptogenesis begins between the dendrites of the spiral ganglia and inner and outer hair cells and progresses in a base-to-apex direction. The number of axons reaches its peak around 20 WG and then decreases to the adult level at 22 WG. As this pruning process occurs, myelination begins in the intra-cochlear portion of CN and extends proximally. By early third trimester, the foetus starts to show physiological responses to vibroacoustic stimuli, and by 29 WG ABRs can be elicited consistently albeit with stronger and slower stimuli.

3.3   Cochlear Nerve Deficiency

There are two possible pathophysiological mechanisms that may lead to CND: one is complete (aplasia) or partial (hypoplasia) failure in development and the other is post-developmental degeneration. Based on the current understanding of CN morphogenesis, associated factors that may provide some insight include the presence or absence of concomitant inner ear anomalies and/or IAC malformations.

Individuals with congenital CND are significantly more likely to have other labyrinthine anomalies than those without CND [3, 25, 34, 35]. This is not surprising, given that the otocyst gives rise to the cochlea, vestibule, semi-circular canals and endolymphatic sac as well as the vestibulocochlear ganglion. It is therefore plausible that developmental arrest occurring early in the embryonic life would likely lead to CND associated with other congenital inner ear malformations. As has been alluded to earlier, migration, growth and survival of vestibulocochlear ganglion cells require expression of various neurotrophic factors by the otocyst [22, 23, 36], which could explain the high prevalence of inner ear dysplasia in CND. In contrast, it appears that the inner ear development is not dependent on neuronal stimulus or trophic effect [37–39]. It is therefore possible that a disturbance in the trophic effect the cochlea exerts on CN neurons may lead to CND as an isolated finding in the presence of a normally developed cochlea [34, 40].

Another potential indicator to be considered is the size of IAC, which is related to migrating VCN neurons and chondrogenesis in the surrounding mesenchyme. IAC stenosis accounts for about 12% of all congenital temporal bone malformations [19]. Until it became possible to actually visualise CN on MRI, the finding of IAC stenosis on computed tomography (CT) was thought to indicate VCN aplasia and therefore considered an absolute contraindication to cochlear implantation [41, 42]. Subsequent studies, however, have demonstrated that a stenotic IAC may contain a hypoplastic CN or functional CN fibres travelling with other nerves within IAC [1, 34, 43]. Conversely, CND in association with normal calibre IAC has also been reported [1, 35, 44]; as the development of IAC commences at 9 WG and is completed by 5 months of gestation, such cases may represent either isolated CN agenesis (vascular insufficiency, uncontrolled apoptosis regulation) or post-developmental degeneration of the nerve (perinatal, neurotrophic viral infections) [35].

A subject that merits discussion in this chapter is auditory neuropathy spectrum disorder (ANSD). ANSD is a heterogeneous group of conditions characterised by marked discrepancy between cochlear and neural functions in the auditory system. The most widely accepted diagnostic criterion is absent or abnormal ABR in association with normal outer hair cell function as evidenced by present cochlear microphonics and/or otoacoustic emissions. It has been estimated that ANSD may account for up to 10–15 % of newly diagnosed cases of hearing loss in children [45, 46]. The prevalence of CND in ANSD is reported to be as high as 18–28 %, compared to 6–16 % in children with SNHL not diagnosed as ANSD [35, 47–49]. Conversely, over 70 % of children with CND have been found to have the audiometric features of ANSD [35, 50]. Although the lesion responsible for dyschrony may be within the inner hair cells (presynaptic) or neural elements (postsynaptic), it appears that, in some children, the ANSD phenotype may result from an absent or hypoplastic CN, especially when there are no medical or familial risk factors identified [35].

Finally, it would be prudent to reflect on some of the potential implications of finding an abnormal CN. The term "cochlear nerve deficiency" is widely used to refer collectively to aplasia and hypoplasia of the nerve. However, some degree of caution is required when using this terminology or interpreting outcomes of studies on the subject. First of all, in the clinical context of profound SNHL, CN aplasia describes a situation where the nerve is not visualised on MRI and is not a histopathological diagnosis. It does not necessarily mean that there is complete absence of nerve fibres or function. Even in the absence of a radiologically visible CN, activation of the primary auditory cortex has been observed on functional MRI [51]. Furthermore, limited benefits from cochlear implantation have been reported in some cases [43, 52, 53]. It has been hypothesised that, in such circumstances, the CN fibres may be travelling with the facial or vestibular nerves [34, 50, 51, 53]. It is therefore important that any radiological finding should be interpreted in conjunction with the audiological profile, in particular behavioural responses to auditory stimuli, and electrophysiological testing if/where appropriate. Second of all, there are a number of different radiological criteria in use for determining what is considered to be a hypoplastic CN. It should be borne in mind that all classifications are based on comparison to a neighbouring nerve, namely, either the facial nerve or one of the branches of the vestibular nerve, rather than a range of absolute values of the nerve diameter. Moreover, by definition of these criteria, some individuals with normal hearing will be deemed to have a hypoplastic nerve radiologically. Third of all, a number of studies have reported a significant difference between outcomes of cochlear implantation between aplastic and hypoplastic CN cases [3, 54]. It is therefore important that, when discussing the subject of CND and particularly outcomes of any intervention, diagnostic criteria used are clearly defined and distinction is made between aplastic (invisible) and hypoplastic (visible but small) CN.

3.4   Conclusion

CN morphogenesis is a complex process involving cell populations from two disparate progenitors, developing in tandem and interacting with each other throughout.
It also requires trophic influence and support from the developing cochlea for proliferation, migration and synaptogenesis. With advancements in auditory implantation and cross-sectional imaging techniques, there is increasing appreciation of the
potential clinical implications and ontogeny of CN. Current research areas of interest include the mechanisms behind determination and delineation of ganglion cell
precursors in the developing otocyst and the formation of synaptic connections with
tonotopically arranged inner and outer hair cells. It is hoped that better understanding of the embryological development of CN will not only lead to further refinement
of auditory implant candidacy but also open doors to regeneration therapies such as
stem cell therapy in the future.

References

1. Adunka OF, Roush PA, Teagle HFB, Brown CJ, Zdanski CJ, Jewells V, et al. Internal auditory canal morphology in children with cochlear nerve deficiency. Otol Neurotol. 2006;27(6):793–801.
2. McClay JE, Booth TN, Parry DA, Johnson R, Roland P. Evaluation of pediatric sensorineural hearing loss with magnetic resonance imaging. Arch Otolaryngol Head Neck Surg. 2008;134(9):945–52. doi:10.1001/archotol.134.9.945.
3. Wu CM, Lee LA, Chen CK, Chan KC, Tsou YT, Ng SH. Impact of cochlear nerve deficiency determined using 3-dimensional magnetic resonance imaging on hearing outcome in children with cochlear implants. Otol Neurotol. 2015;36(1):14–21. doi:10.1097/MAO.0000000000000568.
4. Rosenbluth J. The fine structure of acoustic ganglia in the rat. J Cell Biol. 1962;12:329–59.
5. Harrison RG. Neuroblast versus sheath cell in the development of peripheral nerves. J Comp Neurol. 1924;37:123–205.
6. Yntema CL. An experimental study on the origin of the sensory neurones and sheath cells of the IXth and Xth cranial nerves in Amblystoma punctatum. J Exp Zool. 1943;92:93–119.
7. D'Amico-Martel A, Noden D. Contributions of placodal and neural crest cells to avian cranial peripheral ganglia. Am J Anat. 1983;166:445–68.
8. Fekete DM, Wu DK. Revisiting cell fate specification in the inner ear. Curr Opin Neurobiol. 2002;12:35–42.
9. Barald KF, Kelley MW. From placode to polarization: new tunes in inner ear development. Development. 2004;131:4119–30.
10. Breuskin I, Bodson M, Thelen N, Thiry M, Borgs L, Nguyen L, et al. Glial but not neuronal development in the cochleo-vestibular ganglion requires Sox10. J Neurochem. 2010;114:1827–39. doi:10.1111/j.1471-4159.2010.06897.x.
11. Freyer L, Aggarwal V, Morrow BE. Dual embryonic origin of the mammalian otic vesicle forming the inner ear. Development. 2011;138:5403–14. doi:10.1242/dev.069849.
12. Sandell LL, Butler Tjaden NE, Barlow AJ, Trainor PA. Cochleovestibular nerve development is integrated with migratory neural crest cells. Dev Biol. 2014;385(2):200–10. doi:10.1016/j.ydbio.2013.11.009.

13. O'Rahilly R. The early development of the otic vesicle in staged human embryos. J Embryol Exp Morphol. 1963;11:741–55.
14. Ladher RK, O'Neill P, Begbie J. From shared lineage to distinct functions: the development of the inner ear and epibranchial placodes. Development. 2010;137(11):1777–85. doi:10.1242/dev.040055.
15. Chen J, Streit A. Induction of the inner ear: stepwise specification of otic fate from multipotent progenitors. Hear Res. 2013;297:3–12. doi:10.1016/j.heares.2012.11.018.
16. Cooper ERA. The development of the human auditory pathway from the cochlear ganglion to the medial geniculate body. Acta Anat (Basel). 1948;5(1–2):99–122.
17. Altman J, Bayer S. Development of the cranial nerve ganglia and related nuclei in the rat. Berlin: Springer; 1982.
18. Moore JK, Linthicum Jr FH. The human auditory system: a timeline of development. Int J Audiol. 2007;46:460–78.
19. Li Y, Yang J, Liu J, Wu H. Restudy of malformations of the internal auditory meatus, cochlear nerve canal and cochlear nerve. Eur Arch Otorhinolaryngol. 2015;272(7):1587–96. doi:10.1007/s00405-014-2951-4.
20. Pujol R, Lavigne-Rebillard M. Early stages of innervation and sensory cell differentiation in the human organ of Corti. Acta Otolaryngol Suppl. 1985;423:43–50.
21. Fritzsch B, Silos-Santiago I, Bianchi LM, Fariñas I. The role of neurotrophic factors in regulating the development of inner ear innervation. Trends Neurosci. 1997;20:159–64.
22. Bernd P. The role of neurotrophins during early development. Gene Expr. 2008;14:241–50.
23. Rubel EW, Fritzsch B. Auditory system development: primary auditory neurons and their targets. Annu Rev Neurosci. 2002;25:51–101.
24. McPhee JR, Van De Water TR. Epithelial-mesenchymal tissue interactions guiding otic capsule formation: the role of the otocyst. J Embryol Exp Morphol. 1986;97:1–24.
25. Glastonbury CM, Davidson HC, Harnsberger HR, Butler J, Kertesz TR, Shelton C. Imaging findings of cochlear nerve deficiency. AJNR Am J Neuroradiol. 2002;23:635–43.
26. Lavigne-Rebillard M, Pujol R. Hair cell innervation in the fetal human cochlea. Acta Otolaryngol. 1988;105(5–6):398–402.
27. Ray B, Roy TS, Wadhwa S, Roy KK. Development of the human fetal cochlear nerve: a morphometric study. Hear Res. 2005;202(1–2):74–86.
28. Moore JK, Linthicum Jr FH. Myelination of the human auditory nerve: different time courses for Schwann cell and glial myelin. Ann Otol Rhinol Laryngol. 2001;110:655–61.
29. Birnholz JC, Benecerraf BR. The development of human fetal hearing. Science. 1983;222(4623):516–8.
30. Kuhlman KA, Burns KA, Depp R, Sabbagha RE. Ultrasonic imaging of normal fetal response to external vibratory acoustic stimulation. Am J Obstet Gynecol. 1988;158(1):47–51.
31. Starr A, Amlie RN, Martin WH, Sanders S. Development of auditory function in newborn infants revealed by auditory brainstem potentials. Pediatrics. 1977;60(6):831–9.
32. Krumholz A, Felix JK, Goldstein PH, McKenzie E. Maturation of the brainstem auditory evoked potentials in premature infants. Electroencephalogr Clin Neurophysiol. 1985;62(2):124–34.
33. Hafner H, Pratt H, Blazer S, Snjov P. Critical ages in brainstem development revealed by neonatal 3-channel Lissajous' trajectory of auditory brainstem evoked potentials. Hear Res. 1993;66(2):157–68.
34. Casselman JW, Offeciers FE, Govaerts PJ, Kuhweide R, Geldof H, Somers T, et al. Aplasia and hypoplasia of the vestibulocochlear nerve: diagnosis with MR imaging. Radiology. 1997;202:773–81.
35. Buchman CA, Roush PA, Teagle HFB, Brown CJ, Zdanski CJ, Grose JH. Auditory neuropathy characteristics in children with cochlear nerve deficiency. Ear Hear. 2006;27:399–408.
36. Hossain WA, Brumwell CL, Morest DK. Sequential interactions of fibroblast growth factor-2, brain-derived neurotrophic factor, neurotrophin-3, and their receptors define critical periods in the development of cochlear ganglion cells. Exp Neurol. 2002;175:138–51.

37. Van De Water TR. Effects of removal of the statoacoustic ganglion complex upon the growing otocyst. Ann Otol Rhinol Laryngol. 1976;85:2–31.
38. Corwin JT, Cotanche DA. Development of location-specific hair cell stereocilia in denervated embryonic ears. J Comp Neurol. 1989;288(4):529–37.
39. Nelson EG, Hinojosa R. Aplasia of the cochlear nerve: a temporal bone study. Otol Neurotol. 2001;22(6):790–5.
40. Lefebvre PP, Leprince P, Weber T, Rigo JM, Delree P, Moonen G. Neuronotrophic effect of developing otic vesicle on cochleo-vestibular neurons: evidence for nerve growth factor involvement. Brain Res. 1990;507(2):254–60.
41. Jackler RK, Luxford WM, House WF. Sound detection with the cochlear implant in five ears of four children with congenital malformations of the cochlea. Laryngoscope. 1987;97(3 Pt 2 Suppl 40):15–7.
42. Shelton C, Luxford WM, Tonokawa LL, Lo WW, House WF. The narrow internal auditory canal in children: a contraindication to cochlear implants. Otolaryngol Head Neck Surg. 1989;100:227–31.
43. Govaerts PJ, Casselman J, Daemers K, De Beukelaer C, Yperman M, De Ceulaer G. Cochlear implants in aplasia and hypoplasia of the cochleovestibular nerve. Otol Neurotol. 2003;24:887–91.
44. Yan F, Li J, Xian J, Wang Z, Mo L. The cochlear nerve canal and internal auditory canal in children with normal cochlea but cochlear nerve deficiency. Acta Radiol. 2013;54(3):292–8.
45. Tang TP, McPherson B, Yuen KC, Wong LL, Lee JS. Auditory neuropathy/auditory dys-synchrony in school children with hearing loss: frequency of occurrence. Int J Pediatr Otorhinolaryngol. 2004;68:175Y83.
46. Berlin CI, Hood LJ, Morlet T, Wilensky D, Li L, Mattingly KR, et al. Multi-site diagnosis and management of 260 patients with auditory neuropathy/dys-synchrony (auditory neuropathy spectrum disorder). Int J Audiol. 2010;49(1):30–43.
47. Roche JP, Huang BY, Castillo M, Bassim MK, Adunka OF, Buchman CA. Imaging characteristics of children with auditory neuropathy spectrum disorder. Otol Neurotol. 2010;31:780–8.
48. Walton J, Gibson WP, Sanli H, Prelog K. Predicting cochlear implant outcomes in children with auditory neuropathy. Otol Neurotol. 2008;29:302–9.
49. Huang BY, Roche JP, Buchman CA, Castillo M. Brain stem and inner ear abnormalities in children with auditory neuropathy spectrum disorder and cochlear nerve deficiency. AJNR Am J Neuroradiol. 2010;31(10):1972–9.
50. Levi J, Ames J, Bacik K, Drake C, Morlet T, O'Reilly RC. Clinical characteristics of children with cochlear nerve dysplasias. Laryngoscope. 2013;123(3):752–6. doi:10.1002/lary.23636.
51. Thai-Van H, Fraysse B, Berry I, Berges C, Deguine O, Honegger A, et al. Functional magnetic resonance imaging may avoid misdiagnosis of cochleovestibular nerve aplasia in congenital deafness. Am J Otol. 2000;21:663–70.
52. Zanetti D, Guida M, Barezzani MG, Campovecchi C, Nassif N, Pinelli L, et al. Favorable outcome of cochlear implant in VIIIth nerve deficiency. Otol Neurotol. 2006;27:815–23.
53. Kutz Jr JW, Lee KH, Isaacson B, Booth TN, Sweeney MH, Roland PS. Cochlear implantation in children with cochlear nerve absence or deficiency. Otol Neurotol. 2011;32:956–61.
54. Birman CS, Powell HR, Gibson WP, Elliott EJ. Cochlear implant outcomes in cochlea nerve aplasia and hypoplasia. Otol Neurotol. 2016;37(5):438–45. doi:10.1097/MAO.0000000000000997.

Chapter 4
Morphology, Development, and Neurotrophic Regulation of Cochlear Afferent Innervation

Kenji Kondo, Yulian Jin, Makoto Kinoshita, Tatsuya Yamasoba, and Kimitaka Kaga

Abstract Spiral ganglion neurons (SGNs) are primary sensory neurons of the auditory system that send auditory information encoded by the inner ear to the central nervous system. The success of cochlear implant therapy is totally dependent on the status of SGN function. Therefore, information regarding the neurogenesis, survival, and neurite growth of SGNs is important not only to understand the pathophysiology of sensorineural hearing loss but also to improve cochlear implant therapy. SGNs are anatomically and functionally divided into two subtypes, type I and type II. Type I SGNs connecting inner hair cells contribute to the transmission of sound information into the central auditory pathway, while type II SGNs connecting outer hair cells are involved in active tuning of frequency in the cochlea. In the developing cochlea, the survival and neurite formation of SGNs are strongly regulated by neurotrophic factors, especially neurotrophin 3 (NT-3) and brain-derived neurotrophic factor (BDNF). Also, in the adult cochlea, the loss of hair cells induces secondary loss of SGNs presumably because of a loss of neurotrophic support. When the deafened ear is treated with exogenous BDNF or NT3, there is a significant enhancement of SGN survival and resprouting of neurites. Therefore, chronic application of neurotrophic factors in the cochlea may improve the efficacy of cochlear implants.

Keywords Spiral ganglion neuron • Survival • NT-3 • BDNF

K. Kondo (✉) • M. Kinoshita • T. Yamasoba
Department of Otorhinolaryngology and Head and Neck Surgery, Graduate School
of Medicine, The University of Tokyo, 7-3-1 Hongo, Bunkyo-ku, Tokyo 113-8655, Japan
e-mail: kondok-tky@umin.ac.jp

Y. Jin
Department of Otorhinolaryngology, Yanbian University Hospital,
No.1327, Juzi Street, Yanji 133 000, Republic of China

K. Kaga
National Institute of Sensory Organs, National Tokyo Medical Center,
2-5-1 Higashigaoka, Meguro-Ku, Tokyo 152-8902, Japan

Center for Speech and Hearing Disorders, International University of Health
and Welfare Clinic, 2600-6 Kitakanemaru, Ohtawara, Tochigi 324-0011, Japan

© Springer Science+Business Media Singapore 2017   29
K. Kaga (ed.), *Cochlear Implantation in Children with Inner Ear Malformation
and Cochlear Nerve Deficiency*, Modern Otology and Neurotology,
DOI 10.1007/978-981-10-1400-0_4

4.1 Introduction

Spiral ganglion neurons (SGNs) are primary sensory neurons of the auditory system that send auditory information encoded by the inner ear to the central nervous system. SGNs are bipolar, with a peripheral neurite that forms a synapse with hair cells in the organ of Corti and a central neurite that projects to the cochlear nucleus of the medulla. Corresponding to the precise structural organization of the organ of Corti, the SGNs and their neurites form specific neural circuits along the longitudinal and radial axis of the cochlea to discriminate acoustic signals.

The majority of sensorineural hearing loss is related primarily to the loss of cochlear hair cells. When patients have congenital or acquired profound deafness that cannot be compensated by the use of a hearing aid, they are candidates for cochlear implantation. The success of cochlear implant therapy is totally dependent on the status of SGN function. Therefore, information regarding the neurogenesis, survival, and neurite growth of SGNs is important not only to understand the pathophysiology of the sensorineural hearing loss but also to improve cochlear implant therapy.

In this chapter, we focus on the morphology of SGNs and their development during embryonic and postnatal periods. We also review recent articles regarding the regulation of development and survival of SGNs by neurotrophic factors and their therapeutic potential in cochlear implant therapy. Excellent reviews have recently been published regarding these topics, and the reader is referred to those for more comprehensive information [1–5].

4.2 Morphology of SGNs and Their Neural Connection

The cell body of SGNs is housed in Rosenthal's canal of the cochlea (Fig. 4.1). The total number of SGNs in each cochlea is approximately 32,000–49,000 in humans [6–8] and 13,000–20,000 in rats [9, 10]. Their peripheral neurites pass through the habenula perforata and reach the organ of Corti, which then connect to the inner and outer hair cells. The central neurites extend through the internal auditory canal and project into the cochlear nucleus in the medulla.

SGNs are anatomically and functionally divided into two subtypes, type I and type II. Type I SGNs occupy 90–95 % of all SGNs and have a large cell body, and their central neurites are thicker than peripheral neurites. The peripheral neurites of type I SGNs are ensheathed by peripheral-type myelin of Schwann cells. The central neurites are ensheathed by Schwann cells and by the central-type myelin of oligodendrocytes along their proximal (near the cell body of SGNs) and distal (near the brainstem) portion, respectively (Fig. 4.2). Type II SGNs comprise 5–10 % of all SGNs and have a smaller cell body. Their central and peripheral neurites are approximately the same thickness, and the peripheral neurites are unmyelinated [11–17]. Type I and II SGNs can be differentiated by their immunostaining pattern

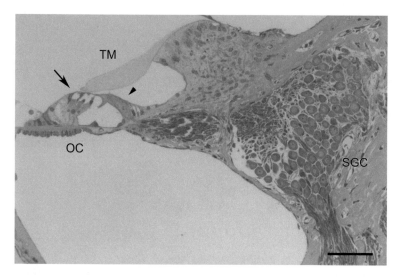

Fig. 4.1 Structure of the cochlea. A semi-thin plastic section through the cochlea of a 2-month-old rat. *OC* organ of Corti, *TM* tectorial membrane, *SGN* spiral ganglion neuron. Scale bar = 0.1 mm (Adapted from Ref. [119] with permission)

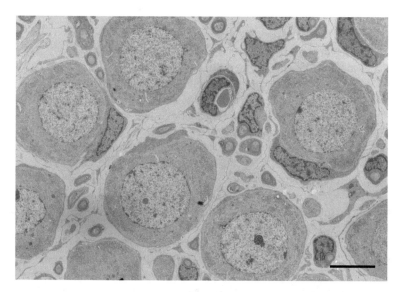

Fig. 4.2 A transmission electron micrograph of SGNs from a 2-month-old rat. SGNs are ensheathed by Schwann cells. *Scale bar = 5 μm*

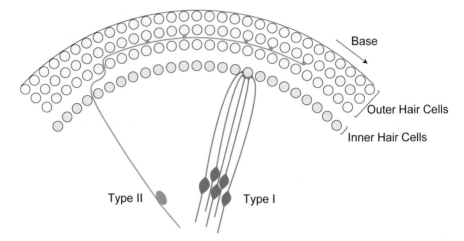

Fig. 4.3 Schematic drawing demonstrating the afferent neural connection in the cochlea. Peripheral neurites of type I SGNs extend from the modiolus toward the organ of Corti in a radial fashion, and each makes synaptic contact with a single inner hair cell. Individual inner hair cells receive multiple projections from type I SGNs. Peripheral neurites of type II SGNs initially extend toward the organ of Corti in a similar manner as type I SGNs. After passing under the row of IHCs, each neurite changes direction in a spiral fashion parallel to an OHC row and forms a synapse with an outer hair cell

for the intermediate filament protein peripherin in mice and rats [18, 19]. The most important anatomical and functional difference between type I and II SGNs is the mode of connection of their peripheral neurites to hair cells (Fig. 4.3). Peripheral neurites of type I SGNs extend from the modiolus toward the organ of Corti in a radial fashion, and each of them makes synaptic contact with a single inner hair cell. Individual inner hair cells receive projections from 10 to 20 processes of type I SGNs. Peripheral neurites of the type II SGNs initially extend toward the organ of Corti in a similar manner as type I SGNs. After passing under the row of inner hair cells, each neurite changes direction in a spiral fashion parallel to an outer hair cell row and forms synapses on approximately three to ten outer hair cells [20–22]. Type I SGNs connecting to inner hair cells contribute to the transmission of sound information into the central auditory pathway, while type II SGNs that connect to outer hair cells are involved in active tuning of frequency in the cochlea [23–25].

The central neurites of type I and II SGNs pass through the internal auditory canal together with the superior vestibular, inferior vestibular, and facial nerves and reach the medulla, where they branch. The short anterior branches project to the ventral cochlear nucleus, and the long posterior branches reach to the dorsal cochlear nucleus [26, 27].

4.3   Development of SGNs

4.3.1   Neurogenesis

The first morphological sign of inner ear development is ectodermal thickening on both sides of the hindbrain, called the otic placode. The placode invaginates and pinches off the surface to become an epithelial vesicle called the otocyst. Otocyst formation occurs at 4 weeks of gestation in humans [28, 29] and embryonic 9.5 days in mice [30–32]. The otocyst undergoes complex shape changes, such as outward extrusion of the duct and epithelial fusion of the cyst wall, and then finally forms a membranous labyrinth consisting of three semicircular canals, the utricle, the saccule, the endolymphatic duct, and the cochlear duct [28–30, 33–36]. In mice, a cell group of future cochleovestibular ganglion can be differentiated at embryonic 10.5 days [37]. The origin of SGNs and whether they are derived from the otocyst or neural crest has long been controversial. An experimental study using chick-quail transplantation [38], as well as a very recent study to trace neural crest cells using a reporter gene [37], clarified that they are basically derived from the otocyst. On the other hand, a recent genetic fate-mapping study reports that SGNs have dual origin and are derived from the otocyst and neural crest [39].

The final cell division in the mouse spiral ganglion occurs at embryonic days 12–16 in mice [40]. After the final cell division, immature SGNs start differentiating and begin to extend central and peripheral neurites. Peripheral neurites penetrate into the organ of Corti at 9 weeks of gestation in humans [41] and embryonic day 11.5 in the mouse [42–44]. The projection of central axons into the cochlear nucleus is slightly later than the projection of peripheral axons into the organ of Corti [14].

4.3.2   Cell Death in SGNs

Studies in gerbils and rats have revealed that the number of SGNs in embryonic periods is approximately 20–30 % larger than that in adults. Neuronal number then decreases within a restricted postnatal time window (first postnatal week in both gerbils and rats) and becomes almost constant thereafter [45, 46]. Apoptosis of SGNs is upregulated corresponding to this period, suggesting that excessive SGNs are eliminated by neuronal cell death [47]. This regulation in neuronal number coincides with the postnatal refinement of cochlear afferent innervation [21, 22, 48]. The current hypothesis explains that SGNs are initially overproduced and that neurons compete with each other to contact their target (i.e., hair cells). The SGNs that have achieved the connection to hair cells are selected and survive, while SGNs that fail to establish a connection undergo apoptosis. Such a selection system is well known in the development of the nervous system to establish a mature innervation pattern [49, 50]. As described in Sect. 4.4, neurotrophic factors provided by hair cells appear to be deeply involved in this process.

4.3.3   Postnatal Rearrangement of Cochlear Afferent Innervation

Initial synaptic contact between hair cells and the peripheral neurites of SGNs in the embryonic period is subsequently remodeled to form their final neural circuit. Studies in gerbils and mice using axonal tracing and immunohistochemistry for type II SGN-specific peripherin have revealed that each afferent fiber of SGNs has contact with both inner and outer hair cells at birth. Most of the type I fibers then eliminate the contact with outer hair cells and retract to the inner hair cell region, while a small number of type II afferent fibers extend to form spiral fibers [21, 22]. The widespread arbors of type I fibers between inner hair cells undergo extensive pruning during this period, and each fiber finally has a synaptic contact with a single inner hair cell [21]. A study on rat SGNs suggested that a similar remodeling of afferent fibers begins around postnatal day (P)3–6 [48]. Interestingly, the expression of the brain-derived neurotrophic factor (BDNF) in the cochlear sensory epithelium, which disappears in the early postnatal period [48, 51], temporarily reappears at P6–P7 in hair and supporting cells [48]. In vitro studies have demonstrated that survival and neurite formation of SGNs in this developmental stage are supported predominantly by BDNF [52, 53]. Therefore, BDNF may play an important role in the rearrangement of innervation patterns of SGNs [48].

4.4   Neurotrophic Factors and SGNs

4.4.1   Expression of Neurotrophins and Their Receptors in the Cochlea

In many developing motor and sensory nervous systems, the establishment of neural circuits is strongly regulated by target-derived neurotrophic factors through the control of cell survival/death and neurite extension. The most well-characterized neurotrophic factors are members of the nerve growth factor (NGF) family of proteins [54, 55]. Four members of this family have been identified in mammals: nerve growth factor (NGF), BDNF, neurotrophin-3 (NT-3), and neurotrophin-4/5 (NT-4/5). These molecules exert their effects on neurons through binding to their high-affinity receptors, members of the Trk family of receptor tyrosine kinases, TrkA, TrkB, and TrkC [56, 57]. The most well-known effect of neurotrophins is the enhancement of neuronal survival [54, 58–60], but a number of studies have elucidated multiple roles of these molecules on neuronal development, including the extension and morphogenesis of neurites [61–69].

In the developing auditory system, in situ hybridization and immunohistochemical studies revealed that BDNF and NT-3 are expressed in the organ of Corti, the target for SGNs [48, 51, 70–74]. At the same time, SGNs express their respective high-affinity neurotrophin receptors, TrkB and TrkC (Fig. 4.4) [59, 71–79].

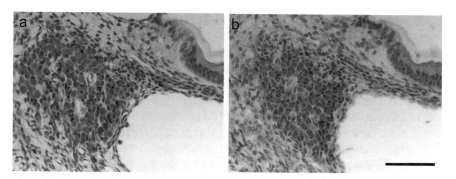

Fig. 4.4 Expression of TrkB and TrkC in the rat cochlea. Paraffin sections from a 5-day-old rat cochlea were immunostained with rabbit polyclonal anti-TrkB (**a**) and anti-TrkC (**b**) antibodies. All SGNs express both TrkB and TrkC (Adapted from Ref. [120] with permission)

Detailed analysis of NT-3 and BDNF expression in mice along the apex-base axis has demonstrated that there is a gradient of expression within the cochlea for each neurotrophin during development [76]. In the early embryonic stage (embryonic day 12.5), BDNF expression is restricted to the apex of the cochlea, and expression spreads toward the basal cochlea later in development. In contrast, NT-3 expression is more confined to the middle and basal turn of the cochlea in the early stages of development, and the expression progresses toward the apex. Expression of both NT-3 and BDNF extends throughout the cochlea longitudinally by embryonic day 16.5 [76], implying that both neurotrophins are available to SGNs that have already come in contact with hair cells through their neurites. NT-3 is more strongly expressed than BDNF [51, 71, 76] and is distributed more widely in the sensory epithelium; both hair cells and supporting cells express NT-3, while BDNF is more restricted to hair cells during this stage [51, 76]. NT-3 continues to be expressed in inner hair cells and adjacent supporting cells of the postnatal and adult cochlea [80], while the expression of BDNF basically disappears in the cochlea [71, 72].

4.4.2 Neurotrophic Support for SGN Survival in Embryonic Development

Knockout mice null for the NT-3 or TrkC gene show considerably reduced numbers of SGNs at birth [81–83]. In contrast, BDNF or TrkB mutant mice mainly lose vestibular neurons [82, 83]. BDNF/NT-3 or TrkB/TrkC double homozygous mutants lose all cochlear and vestibular neurons around birth [83, 84].

More detailed analysis along the apex-base axis of the cochlea revealed that NT-3 knockout mice show an almost complete loss of innervation in the basal turns with a more mild decrease in innervation in the middle and apical turns [81]. In contrast, BDNF-deficient mice demonstrate mild loss of SGNs primarily in the apical turns [85]. These phenotypic differences in knockout mice would be explained by developmental changes in the expression of NT-3 and BDNF described above. When SGNs reach the critical period where they require neurotrophic support for survival, SGNs in NT-3 null mice are only supported by BDNF expressed in the apical region. Therefore, SGNs at the base of the cochlea die through apoptosis because of a lack of neurotrophic support. Conversely, in BDNF null mice, SGNs at this critical period are only supported by NT-3 expressed in the basal region, resulting in subsequent neuronal death in the apical region. The replacement of the NT-3-coding sequence with that of BDNF almost completely rescues the loss of basal turn SGNs by NT-3 absence [76, 86]. These results suggest that NT-3 and BDNF can be functionally equivalent for the survival of SGNs prenatally, and the specific pattern of neuronal loss in the cochlea of NT-3 and BDNF knockout mice is attributed to the availability of neurotrophic support during the critical period when SGNs need it for survival [76].

4.4.3   Other Neurotrophic Factors Involved in the Development of Cochlear Innervation

Recent studies have demonstrated that neurotrophic factors other than neurotrophins, such as glial cell-derived neurotrophic factor (GDNF) and ciliary neurotrophic factor (CNTF), are also expressed in the auditory system. For example, GDNF is expressed in the postnatal cochlea, and the expression increases concomitant with hearing onset [87, 88], suggesting that GDNF may play a role in the adult function of the cochlea. GDNF promotes survival of SGNs both in vivo [87, 89] and in vitro [87, 90]. CNTF belongs to the interleukin-6 family of cytokines. The expression of CNTF is not only in the cochlea but also in the cochlear nucleus [88]. CNTF promotes SGN survival and neuritogenesis in vitro [91–93].

4.4.4   Neurotrophic Factors Promote Survival and Neuritogenesis of SGNs In Vitro

In vitro studies further support the hypothesis that both NT-3 and BDNF can promote SGN survival and neuritogenesis [59, 70, 73, 78, 79, 91, 94–98]. These studies have suggested that among the neurotrophic factors, BDNF shows the strongest promoting effects of survival and neurite formation on early postnatal SGNs (Fig. 4.5).

We recently examined the age-dependent changes in responsiveness of SGNs to NT-3, BDNF, and leukemia inhibitory factor (LIF) using dissociated cultures [53]. Our data suggest that these neurotrophic factors may predominantly support different ontogenetic events in different developmental stages in the innervation of the inner ear (Figs. 4.6 and 4.7).

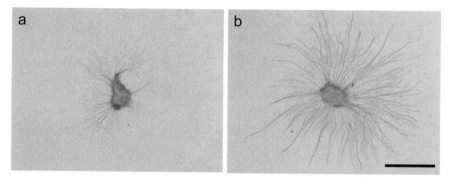

Fig. 4.5 The effect of BDNF on neuritogenesis in 5-day-old rat SGN explants. The explants were cultured for 3 days in media either without neurotrophin (**a**) or supplemented with 10 ng/ml of BDNF (**b**) and then fixed and immunostained with anti-NF200 antibody. The number of neurites sprouting and the length of neurite extension were significantly increased following supplementation with BDNF. Scale bar = 0.5 mm (Adapted from Ref. [119] with permission)

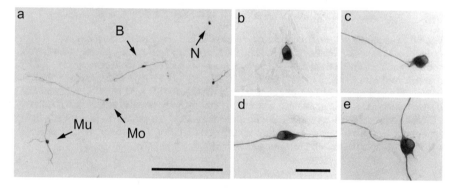

Fig. 4.6 (**a**) An example of cultured SGNs after 12 h in primary growth media containing serum and a further 72 h in serum-free maintenance media. Cells were fixed and immunostained with anti-NF200 antibody. Surviving SGNs were identified as NF200-positive cells. Cultured neurons either had no neurites (indicated as **N**) or were monopolar (indicated as **Mo**; with one neurite emanating from the cell body), bipolar (indicated as **B**; with two neurites emanating from the cell body), or multipolar (indicated as **Mu**; with three or more neurites emanating from the cell body) morphologies. High-magnification views of N, Mo, B, and Mu SGNs shown in (**a**) are in (**b**), (**c**), (**d**), and (**e**), respectively. Scale bars = 0.5 mm in (**a**) and 50 μm in (**b**–**e**) (Adapted from Ref. [53] with permission)

In this analysis, we demonstrated that LIF has a strong effect on neurite extension of postnatal SGNs (Fig. 4.7). LIF is a member of the interleukin-6 family as CNTF and has been reported to enhance neurite extension in a variety of other neuronal types [99, 100]. In particular, recent studies have demonstrated that LIF mediates the enhanced intrinsic growth status after a conditioning lesion [99, 101], suggesting that LIF can play a role in the regeneration of injured neurites. Therefore, our results, together with those in previous reports [92, 93, 97], suggest that the

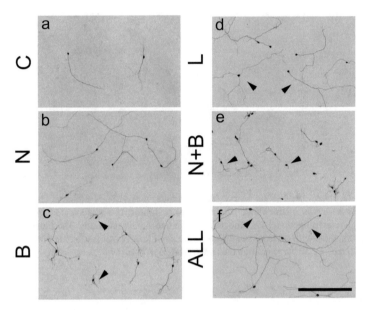

Fig. 4.7 The effects of neurotrophic factors on survival and neuritogenesis in 5-day-old rat SGNs in dissociated cultures. Neurons were cultured for 12 h in serum-containing primary growth media and for a further 72 h in serum-free maintenance media without any neurotrophic factors (**a**; *C*), or supplemented with 50 ng/ml of NT-3 (**b**; *N*), BDNF (**c**; *B*), LIF (**d**; *L*), a combination of NT-3 and BDNF (50 ng/ml each; *N+B*) (**e**), or a combination of NT-3, BDNF, and LIF (50 ng/ml each; *ALL*) (**f**) and then fixed and immunostained with anti-NF200 antibody. Survival effects of NT-3, BDNF, LIF, and their combinations compared with untreated control are shown. The length of neurites appeared to increase following treatment with LIF or *ALL* factors (*arrowheads* in **d**, **f**). *Scale bar* = 0.5 mm (Adapted from Ref. [53] with permission)

application of exogenous LIF, alone or together with neurotrophins, may be clinically valuable as a treatment for central axon injury from trauma or surgical removal of acoustic tumors, as well as for peripheral dendrites to improve the efficacy of cochlear implants.

4.4.5 Damage of the Organ of Corti and Secondary Degeneration of SGNs

In the adult inner ear, hair cells (especially inner hair cells) appear to be the major source of neurotrophic support to SGNs. The loss of hair cells induces secondary loss of SGNs presumably because of a loss in neurotrophic support [88]. In such secondary degenerative processes, the peripheral neurites first retract following hair cell loss, and the degeneration of SGNs occurs in long-term deafness [102]. The speed of degeneration appears to depend on the species; in deafened rats and guinea pigs, SGN death occurs over a few months [103–106], whereas in deafened cats, SGN death occurs over months to years [107]. In humans, SGNs are capable of surviving for many years in the absence of hair cells [108, 109]. The reason underlying this interspecies difference is unclear.

4.4.6 Therapeutic Potential of Neurotrophic Factors in Cochlear Implant Therapy

The degenerative process of SGNs can deteriorate the efficacy of cochlear implants. Therefore, the development of a therapeutic strategy to prevent the degeneration of SGNs is needed. When the deafened ear is treated with exogenous BDNF, NT-3, or other neurotrophic factors, there is a significant enhancement of SGN survival [110–116]. Therefore, chronic application of NTs in the cochlea may have benefits in maintaining the efficacy of cochlear implants. It is interesting that despite the limited endogenous expression of BDNF in the mature adult cochlea, the SGNs retain the capacity to respond to BDNF for survival. This finding agrees with that of our in vitro study, in which rat SGNs harvested from postnatal day 20, when almost all major developmental events for SGNs are complete and hearing function has matured by this age [16], respond to BDNF for survival [53].

Such exogenous neurotrophic factors not only prevent the cell death of deafferentated SGNs but also promote the regrowth of peripheral processes toward a new source of neurotrophic factors that act as chemoattractants [110, 113, 114, 117]. Resprouting of the peripheral neurites of SGNs would enable the reduction of stimulation current, thereby diminishing current spread and improving the number of perceptual channels achieved with cochlear implant electrode arrays. It may also enable the use of CI electrodes that have a larger number of channels.

To deliver neurotrophic factors into the cochlea, intracochlear administration using osmotic pumps and viral vectors has been used to provide trophic factors to the cochlea (for review, see [3, 5]). We recently developed a CI electrode array coated with a biocompatible 2-methacryloyloxyethyl phosphorylcholine (MPC) polymer [118], which is expected to ensure safe and reliable insertion and anti-inflammatory effects. MPC polymers contain extremely hydrophilic phosphorylcholine in their side chains, and surfaces covered with an ultrathin (50 nm) MPC layer have been shown to exhibit good wettability and low friction. MPC polymers have been applied to several medical devices, such as artificial hip joints, implantable blood pumps, cardiovascular stents, oxygenator, and soft contact lenses. One of the potential advantages of using MPC polymer to coat cochlear implant electrodes is that MPC polymer can be a reservoir for various factors, including neurotrophic factors. There is great hope that in the near future, modified MPC polymers that elute such substances will play a key role in enhancing performance after CI.

References

1. Yang T, Kersigo J, Jahan I, Pan N, Fritzsch B. The molecular basis of making spiral ganglion neurons and connecting them to hair cells of the organ of Corti. Hear Res. 2011;278:21–33. doi:10.1016/j.heares.2011.03.002.
2. Delacroix L, Malgrange B. Cochlear afferent innervation development. Hear Res. 2015;330:157–69. doi:10.1016/j.heares.2015.07.015.
3. Ramekers D, Versnel H, Grolman W, Klis SF. Neurotrophins and their role in the cochlea. Hear Res. 2012;288:19–33. doi:10.1016/j.heares.2012.03.002.
4. Green SH, Bailey E, Wang Q, Davis RL. The Trk A, B, C's of neurotrophins in the cochlea. Anat Rec (Hoboken). 2012;295:1877–95. doi:10.1002/ar.22587.
5. Budenz CL, Pfingst BE, Raphael Y. The use of neurotrophin therapy in the inner ear to augment cochlear implantation outcomes. Anat Rec (Hoboken). 2012;295:1896–908. doi:10.1002/ar.22586.
6. Spoendlin H, Schrott A. Quantitative evaluation of the human cochlear nerve. Acta Otolaryngol Suppl. 1990;470:61–70.
7. Ishiyama G, Geiger C, Lopez IA, Ishiyama A. Spiral and vestibular ganglion estimates in archival temporal bones obtained by design based stereology and Abercrombie methods. J Neurosci Methods. 2011;196:76–80. doi:10.1016/j.jneumeth.2011.01.001.
8. Tang Y, Lopez I, Ishiyama A. Application of unbiased stereology on archival human temporal bone. Laryngoscope. 2002;112:526–33. doi:10.1097/00005537-200203000-00022.
9. Hall RD, Massengill JL. The number of primary auditory afferents in the rat. Hear Res. 1997;103:75–84. doi:10.1016/S0378-5955(96)00166-9.
10. Keithley EM, Feldman ML. Spiral ganglion cell counts in an age-graded series of rat cochleas. J Comp Neurol. 1979;188:429–42. doi:10.1002/cne.901880306.
11. Perkins RE, Morest DK. A study of cochlear innervation patterns in cats and rats with the Golgi method and Nomarkski Optics. J Comp Neurol. 1975;163:129–58. doi:10.1002/cne.901630202.
12. Simmons DD, Manson-Gieseke L, Hendrix TW, Morris K, Williams SJ. Postnatal maturation of spiral ganglion neurons: a horseradish peroxidase study. Hear Res. 1991;55:81–91. doi:10.1016/0378-5955(91)90094-P.
13. Toesca A. Central and peripheral myelin in the rat cochlear and vestibular nerves. Neurosci Lett. 1996;221:21–4. doi:10.1016/S0304-3940(96)13273-0.
14. Rubel EW, Fritzsch B. Auditory system development: primary auditory neurons and their targets. Annu Rev Neurosci. 2002;25:51–101. doi:10.1146/annurev.neuro.25.112701.142849.
15. Tang W, Zhang Y, Chang Q, Ahmad S, Dahlke I, Yi H, et al. Connexin29 is highly expressed in cochlear Schwann cells, and it is required for the normal development and function of the auditory nerve of mice. J Neurosci. 2006;26:1991–9. doi:10.1523/JNEUROSCI.5055-05.2006.
16. Pujol R, Lavigne-Rebillard M, Lenoir M. Development of sensory and neural structures in the mammalian cochlea. In: Rubel EW, Popper AN, Fay RR, editors. Development of auditory system. New York: Springer; 1998. p. 146–92.
17. Rusznak Z, Szucs G. Spiral ganglion neurones: an overview of morphology, firing behaviour, ionic channels and function. Pflugers Arch. 2009;457:1303–25. doi.10.1007/s00424-008-0586-2.
18. Barclay M, Ryan AF, Housley GD. Type I vs type II spiral ganglion neurons exhibit differential survival and neuritogenesis during cochlear development. Neural Dev. 2011;6:33. doi:10.1186/1749-8104-6-33.
19. Hafidi A. Peripherin-like immunoreactivity in type II spiral ganglion cell body and projections. Brain Res. 1998;805:181–90. doi:10.1016/S0006-8993(98)00448-X.
20. Berglund AM, Ryugo DK. Hair cell innervation by spiral ganglion neurons in the mouse. J Comp Neurol. 1987;255:560–70. doi:10.1002/cne.902550408.
21. Echteler SM. Developmental segregation in the afferent projections to mammalian auditory hair cells. Proc Natl Acad Sci U S A. 1992;89:6324–7.

22. Huang LC, Thorne PR, Housley GD, Montgomery JM. Spatiotemporal definition of neurite outgrowth, refinement and retraction in the developing mouse cochlea. Development. 2007;134:2925–33. doi:10.1242/dev.001925.
23. Froud KE, Wong AC, Cederholm JM, Klugmann M, Sandow SL, Julien JP, et al. Type II spiral ganglion afferent neurons drive medial olivocochlear reflex suppression of the cochlear amplifier. Nat Commun. 2015;6:7115. doi:10.1038/ncomms8115.
24. Jagger DJ, Housley GD. Membrane properties of type II spiral ganglion neurones identified in a neonatal rat cochlear slice. J Physiol. 2003;552:525–33. doi:10.1113/jphysiol.2003.052589.
25. Thiers FA, Nadol Jr JB, Liberman MC. Reciprocal synapses between outer hair cells and their afferent terminals: evidence for a local neural network in the mammalian cochlea. J Assoc Res Otolaryngol. 2008;9:477–89. doi:10.1007/s10162-008-0135-x.
26. Brown MC, Ledwith 3rd JV. Projections of thin (type-II) and thick (type-I) auditory-nerve fibers into the cochlear nucleus of the mouse. Hear Res. 1990;49:105–18. doi:10.1016/0378-5955(90)90098-A.
27. Morgan YV, Ryugo DK, Brown MC. Central trajectories of type II (thin) fibers of the auditory nerve in cats. Hear Res. 1994;79:74–82. doi:10.1016/0378-5955(94)90128-7.
28. Lim R, Brichta AM. Anatomical and physiological development of the human inner ear. Hear Res. 2016. doi:10.1016/j.heares.2016.02.004.
29. Nishikori T, Hatta T, Kawauchi H, Otani H. Apoptosis during inner ear development in human and mouse embryos: an analysis by computer-assisted three-dimensional reconstruction. Anat Embryol (Berl). 1999;200:19–26. doi:10.1007/s004290050255.
30. Martin P, Swanson GJ. Descriptive and experimental-analysis of the epithelial remodellings that control semicircular canal formation in the developing mouse inner-ear. Dev Biol. 1993;159:549–58. doi:10.1006/dbio.1993.1263.
31. Sher AE. The embryonic and postnatal development of the inner ear of the mouse. Acta Otolaryngol Suppl. 1971;285:1–77. doi:10.3109/00016487109127849.
32. Kikuchi T, Tonosaki A, Takasaka T. Development of apical-surface structures of mouse otic placode. Acta Otolaryngol. 1988;106:200–7. doi:10.3109/00016488809106426.
33. Bissonnette JP, Fekete DM. Standard atlas of the gross anatomy of the developing inner ear of the chicken. J Comp Neurol. 1996;368:620–30. doi:10.1002/(SICI)1096-9861(19960513)368:4<620::AID-CNE12>3.0.CO;2-L.
34. Lang H, Bever MM, Fekete DM. Cell proliferation and cell death in the developing chick inner ear: spatial and temporal patterns. J Comp Neurol. 2000;417:205–20. doi:10.1002/(SICI)1096-9861(20000207)417:2<205::AID-CNE6>3.0.CO;2-Y.
35. Represa JJ, Moro JA, Gato A, Pastor F, Barbosa E. Patterns of epithelial cell death during early development of the human inner ear. Ann Otol Rhinol Laryngol. 1990;99:482–8. doi:10.1177/000348949009900613.
36. Torres M, Giraldez F. The development of the vertebrate inner ear. Mech Dev. 1998;71:5–21. doi:10.1016/S0925-4773(97)00155-X.
37. Sandell LL, Butler Tjaden NE, Barlow AJ, Trainor PA. Cochleovestibular nerve development is integrated with migratory neural crest cells. Dev Biol. 2014;385:200–10. doi:10.1016/j.ydbio.2013.11.009.
38. D'Amico-Martel A, Noden DM. Contributions of placodal and neural crest cells to avian cranial peripheral ganglia. Am J Anat. 1983;166:445–68. doi:10.1002/aja.1001660406.
39. Freyer L, Aggarwal V, Morrow BE. Dual embryonic origin of the mammalian otic vesicle forming the inner ear. Development. 2011;138:5403–14. doi:10.1242/dev.069849.
40. Ruben RJ. Development of the inner ear of the mouse: a radioautographic study of terminal mitoses. Acta Otolaryngol. 1967;220(Suppl:Suppl):1–44. doi:10.3109/00016486709127790.
41. Pechriggl EJ, Bitsche M, Glueckert R, Rask-Andersen H, Blumer MJ, Schrott-Fischer A, et al. Development of the innervation of the human inner ear. Dev Neurobiol. 2015;75:683–702. doi:10.1002/dneu.22242.

42. Matei V, Pauley S, Kaing S, Rowitch D, Beisel KW, Morris K, et al. Smaller inner ear sensory epithelia in Neurog 1 null mice are related to earlier hair cell cycle exit. Dev Dyn. 2005;234:633–50. doi:10.1002/dvdy.20551.

43. Bruce LL, Kingsley J, Nichols DH, Fritzsch B. The development of vestibulocochlear efferents and cochlear afferents in mice. Int J Dev Neurosci. 1997;15:671–92. doi:10.1016/S0736-5748(96)00120-7.

44. Fritzsch B. Development of inner ear afferent connections: forming primary neurons and connecting them to the developing sensory epithelia. Brain Res Bull. 2003;60:423–33.

45. Rueda J, de la Sen C, Juiz JM, Merchan JA. Neuronal loss in the spiral ganglion of young rats. Acta Otolaryngol. 1987;104:417–21. doi:10.3109/00016488709128269.

46. Echteler SM, Nofsinger YC. Development of ganglion cell topography in the postnatal cochlea. J Comp Neurol. 2000;425:436–46. doi:10.1002/1096-9861(20000925)425:3<436::AID-CNE8>3.0.CO;2-1.

47. Echteler SM, Magardino T, Rontal M. Spatiotemporal patterns of neuronal programmed cell death during postnatal development of the gerbil cochlea. Brain Res Dev Brain Res. 2005;157:192–200. doi:10.1016/j.devbrainres.2005.04.004.

48. Wiechers B, Gestwa G, Mack A, Carroll P, Zenner HP, Knipper M. A changing pattern of brain-derived neurotrophic factor expression correlates with the rearrangement of fibers during cochlear development of rats and mice. J Neurosci. 1999;19:3033–42.

49. Pettmann B, Henderson CE. Neuronal cell death. Neuron. 1998;20:633–47. doi:10.1016/S0896-6273(00)81004-1.

50. Oppenheim RW. Cell death during development of the nervous system. Annu Rev Neurosci. 1991;14:453–501. doi:10.1146/annurev.ne.14.030191.002321.

51. Wheeler EF, Bothwell M, Schecterson LC, von Bartheld CS. Expression of BDNF and NT-3 mRNA in hair cells of the organ of Corti: quantitative analysis in developing rats. Hear Res. 1994;73:46–56. doi:10.1016/0378-5955(94)90281-X.

52. Kondo K, Pak K, Chavez E, Mullen L, Euteneuer S, Ryan AF. Changes in responsiveness of rat spiral ganglion neurons to neurotrophins across age: differential regulation of survival and neuritogenesis. Int J Neurosci. 2013;123:465–75. doi:10.3109/00207454.2013.764497.

53. Jin Y, Kondo K, Ushio M, Kaga K, Ryan AF, Yamasoba T. Developmental changes in the responsiveness of rat spiral ganglion neurons to neurotrophic factors in dissociated culture: differential responses for survival, neuritogenesis and neuronal morphology. Cell Tissue Res. 2013;351:15–27. doi:10.1007/s00441-012-1526-1.

54. Snider WD. Functions of the neurotrophins during nervous system development: what the knockouts are teaching us. Cell. 1994;77:627–38. doi:10.1016/0092-8674(94)90048-5.

55. Levi-Montalcini R. The nerve growth factor 35 years later. Science. 1987;237:1154–62. doi:10.1126/science.3306916.

56. Huang EJ, Reichardt LF. Trk receptors: roles in neuronal signal transduction. Annu Rev Biochem. 2003;72:609–42. doi:10.1146/annurev.biochem.72.121801.161629.

57. Friedman WJ, Greene LA. Neurotrophin signaling via Trks and p75. Exp Cell Res. 1999;253:131–42. doi:10.1006/excr.1999.4705.

58. Barde YA. Trophic factors and neuronal survival. Neuron. 1989;2:1525–34. doi:10.1016/0896-6273(89)90040-8.

59. Mou K, Hunsberger CL, Cleary JM, Davis RL. Synergistic effects of BDNF and NT-3 on postnatal spiral ganglion neurons. J Comp Neurol. 1997;386:529–39. doi:10.1002/(SICI)1096-9861(19971006)386:4<529::AID-CNE1>3.0.CO;2-4.

60. Buchman VL, Davies AM. Different neurotrophins are expressed and act in a developmental sequence to promote the survival of embryonic sensory neurons. Development. 1993;118:989–1001.

61. Davies AM. Neurotrophins: neurotrophic modulation of neurite growth. Curr Biol. 2000;10:R198–200. doi:10.1016/S0960-9822(00)00351-1.

62. Cohen-Cory S, Fraser SE. Effects of brain-derived neurotrophic factor on optic axon branching and remodelling in vivo. Nature. 1995;378:192–6. doi:10.1038/378192a0.

63. Segal RA, Pomeroy SL, Stiles CD. Axonal growth and fasciculation linked to differential expression of BDNF and NT3 receptors in developing cerebellar granule cells. J Neurosci. 1995;15:4970–81.

64. Lentz SI, Knudson CM, Korsmeyer SJ, Snider WD. Neurotrophins support the development of diverse sensory axon morphologies. J Neurosci. 1999;19:1038–48.

65. Snider WD. Nerve growth factor enhances dendritic arborization of sympathetic ganglion cells in developing mammals. J Neurosci. 1988;8:2628–34.

66. Kimpinski K, Campenot RB, Mearow K. Effects of the neurotrophins nerve growth factor, neurotrophin-3, and brain-derived neurotrophic factor (BDNF) on neurite growth from adult sensory neurons in compartmented cultures. J Neurobiol. 1997;33:395–410. doi:10.1002/(SICI)1097-4695(199710)33:4<395::AID-NEU5>3.0.CO;2-5.

67. Orike N, Thrasivoulou C, Wrigley A, Cowen T. Differential regulation of survival and growth in adult sympathetic neurons: an in vitro study of neurotrophin responsiveness. J Neurobiol. 2001;47:295–305. doi:10.1002/neu.1036.

68. Scott SA, Davies AM. Age-related effects of nerve growth factor on the morphology of embryonic sensory neurons in vitro. J Comp Neurol. 1993;337:277–85. doi:10.1002/cne.903370208.

69. Ulupinar E, Jacquin MF, Erzurumlu RS. Differential effects of NGF and NT-3 on embryonic trigeminal axon growth patterns. J Comp Neurol. 2000;425:202–18. doi:10.1002/1096-9861(20000918)425:2<202::AID-CNE4>3.0.CO;2-T.

70. Pirvola U, Ylikoski J, Palgi J, Lehtonen E, Arumae U, Saarma M. Brain-derived neurotrophic factor and neurotrophin 3 mRNAs in the peripheral target fields of developing inner ear ganglia. Proc Natl Acad Sci U S A. 1992;89:9915–9. doi:10.1073/pnas.89.20.9915.

71. Schecterson LC, Bothwell M. Neurotrophin and neurotrophin receptor mRNA expression in developing inner ear. Hear Res. 1994;73:92–100. doi:10.1016/0378-5955(94)90286-0.

72. Ylikoski J, Pirvola U, Moshnyakov M, Palgi J, Arumae U, Saarma M. Expression patterns of neurotrophin and their receptor mRNAs in the rat inner ear. Hear Res. 1993;65:69–78. doi:10.1016/0378-5955(93)90202-C.

73. Pirvola U, Arumae U, Moshnyakov M, Palgi J, Saarma M, Ylikoski J. Coordinated expression and function of neurotrophins and their receptors in the rat inner ear during target innervation. Hear Res. 1994;75:131–44. doi:10.1016/0378-5955(94)90064-7.

74. Pirvola U, Hallbook F, Xing-Qun L, Virkkala J, Saarma M, Ylikoski J. Expression of neurotrophins and Trk receptors in the developing, adult, and regenerating avian cochlea. J Neurobiol. 1997;33:1019–33.

75. Knipper M, Zimmermann U, Rohbock K, Kopschall I, Zenner HP. Expression of neurotrophin receptor trkB in rat cochlear hair cells at time of rearrangement of innervation. Cell Tissue Res. 1996;283:339–53. doi:10.1007/s004410050545.

76. Farinas I, Jones KR, Tessarollo L, Vigers AJ, Huang E, Kirstein M, et al. Spatial shaping of cochlear innervation by temporally regulated neurotrophin expression. J Neurosci. 2001;21:6170–80.

77. Cochran SL, Stone JS, Bermingham-McDonogh O, Akers SR, Lefcort F, Rubel EW. Ontogenetic expression of trk neurotrophin receptors in the chick auditory system. J Comp Neurol. 1999;413:271–88. doi:10.1002/(SICI)1096-9861(19991018)413:2<271::AID-CNE8>3.0.CO;2-L.

78. Vazquez E, Van de Water TR, Del Valle M, Vega JA, Staecker H, Giraldez F, et al. Pattern of trkB protein-like immunoreactivity in vivo and the in vitro effects of brain-derived neurotrophic factor (BDNF) on developing cochlear and vestibular neurons. Anat Embryol (Berl). 1994;189:157–67. doi:10.1007/BF00185774.

79. Zheng JI, Stewart RR, Gao WQ. Neurotrophin-4/5 enhances survival of cultured spiral ganglion neurons and protects them from cisplatin neurotoxicity. J Neurosci. 1995;15:5079–87.

80. Sugawara M, Murtie JC, Stankovic KM, Liberman MC, Corfas G. Dynamic patterns of neurotrophin 3 expression in the postnatal mouse inner ear. J Comp Neurol. 2007;501:30–7. doi:10.1002/cne.21227.

81. Fritzsch B, Farinas I, Reichardt LF. Lack of neurotrophin 3 causes losses of both classes of spiral ganglion neurons in the cochlea in a region-specific fashion. J Neurosci. 1997;17:6213–25.

82. Fritzsch B, Barbacid M, Silos-Santiago I. The combined effects of trkB and trkC mutations on the innervation of the inner ear. Int J Dev Neurosci. 1998;16:493–505. doi:10.1016/S0736-5748(98)00043-4.

83. Ernfors P, Van De Water T, Loring J, Jaenisch R. Complementary roles of BDNF and NT-3 in vestibular and auditory development. Neuron. 1995;14:1153–64. doi:10.1016/0896-6273(95)90263-5.

84. Silos-Santiago I, Fagan AM, Garber M, Fritzsch B, Barbacid M. Severe sensory deficits but normal CNS development in newborn mice lacking TrkB and TrkC tyrosine protein kinase receptors. Eur J Neurosci. 1997;9:2045–56. doi:10.1111/j.1460-9568.1997.tb01372.x.

85. Bianchi LM, Conover JC, Fritzsch B, DeChiara T, Lindsay RM, Yancopoulos GD. Degeneration of vestibular neurons in late embryogenesis of both heterozygous and homozygous BDNF null mutant mice. Development. 1996;122:1965–73.

86. Coppola V, Kucera J, Palko ME, Martinez-De Velasco J, Lyons WE, Fritzsch B, et al. Dissection of NT3 functions in vivo by gene replacement strategy. Development. 2001;128:4315–27.

87. Ylikoski J, Pirvola U, Virkkala J, Suvanto P, Liang XQ, Magal E, et al. Guinea pig auditory neurons are protected by glial cell line-derived growth factor from degeneration after noise trauma. Hear Res. 1998;124:17–26. doi:10.1016/S0378-5955(98)00095-1.

88. Bailey EM, Green SH. Postnatal expression of neurotrophic factors accessible to spiral ganglion neurons in the auditory system of adult hearing and deafened rats. J Neurosci. 2014;34:13110–26. doi:10.1523/JNEUROSCI.1014-14.2014.

89. Kanzaki S, Stover T, Kawamoto K, Prieskorn DM, Altschuler RA, Miller JM, et al. Glial cell line-derived neurotrophic factor and chronic electrical stimulation prevent VIII cranial nerve degeneration following denervation. J Comp Neurol. 2002;454:350–60. doi:10.1002/cne.10480.

90. Wei D, Jin Z, Jarlebark L, Scarfone E, Ulfendahl M. Survival, synaptogenesis, and regeneration of adult mouse spiral ganglion neurons in vitro. Dev Neurobiol. 2007;67:108–22. doi:10.1002/dneu.20336.

91. Hartnick CJ, Staecker H, Malgrange B, Lefebvre PP, Liu W, Moonen G, et al. Neurotrophic effects of BDNF and CNTF, alone and in combination, on postnatal day 5 rat acoustic ganglion neurons. J Neurobiol. 1996;30:246–54. doi:10.1002/(SICI)1097-4695(199606)30:2<246::AID-NEU6>3.0.CO;2-5.

92. Vieira M, Christensen BL, Wheeler BC, Feng AS, Kollmar R. Survival and stimulation of neurite outgrowth in a serum-free culture of spiral ganglion neurons from adult mice. Hear Res. 2007;230:17–23. doi:10.1016/j.heares.2007.03.005.

93. Whitlon DS, Grover M, Tristano J, Williams T, Coulson MT. Culture conditions determine the prevalence of bipolar and monopolar neurons in cultures of dissociated spiral ganglion. Neuroscience. 2007;146:833–40. doi:10.1016/j.neuroscience.2007.01.036.

94. Avila MA, Varela-Nieto I, Romero G, Mato JM, Giraldez F, Van De Water TR, et al. Brain-derived neurotrophic factor and neurotrophin-3 support the survival and neuritogenesis response of developing cochleovestibular ganglion neurons. Dev Biol. 1993;159:266–75. doi:10.1006/dbio.1993.1239.

95. Marzella PL, Gillespie LN, Clark GM, Bartlett PF, Kilpatrick TJ. The neurotrophins act synergistically with LIF and members of the TGF-beta superfamily to promote the survival of spiral ganglia neurons in vitro. Hear Res. 1999;138:73–80. doi:10.1016/S0378-5955(99)00152-5.

96. Hegarty JL, Kay AR, Green SH. Trophic support of cultured spiral ganglion neurons by depolarization exceeds and is additive with that by neurotrophins or cAMP and requires elevation of [Ca2+]i within a set range. J Neurosci. 1997;17:1959–70.

97. Gillespie LN, Clark GM, Bartlett PF, Marzella PL. LIF is more potent than BDNF in promoting neurite outgrowth of mammalian auditory neurons in vitro. Neuroreport. 2001;12:275–9.

98. Malgrange B, Lefebvre P, Van de Water TR, Staecker H, Moonen G. Effects of neurotrophins on early auditory neurones in cell culture. Neuroreport. 1996;7:913–7.

99. Cafferty WB, Gardiner NJ, Gavazzi I, Powell J, McMahon SB, Heath JK, et al. Leukemia inhibitory factor determines the growth status of injured adult sensory neurons. J Neurosci. 2001;21:7161–70.

100. Leibinger M, Muller A, Andreadaki A, Hauk TG, Kirsch M, Fischer D. Neuroprotective and axon growth-promoting effects following inflammatory stimulation on mature retinal ganglion cells in mice depend on ciliary neurotrophic factor and leukemia inhibitory factor. J Neurosci. 2009;29:14334–41. doi:10.1523/JNEUROSCI.2770-09.2009.

101. Hyatt Sachs H, Rohrer H, Zigmond RE. The conditioning lesion effect on sympathetic neurite outgrowth is dependent on gp130 cytokines. Exp Neurol. 2010;223:516–22. doi:10.1016/j.expneurol.2010.01.019.

102. Spoendlin H. Retrograde degeneration of the cochlear nerve. Acta Otolaryngol. 1975;79:266–75. doi:10.3109/00016487509124683.

103. Webster M, Webster DB. Spiral ganglion neuron loss following organ of Corti loss: a quantitative study. Brain Res. 1981;212:17–30. doi:10.1016/0006-8993(81)90028-7.

104. Koitchev K, Guilhaume A, Cazals Y, Aran JM. Spiral ganglion changes after massive aminoglycoside treatment in the guinea pig. Counts and ultrastructure. Acta Otolaryngol. 1982;94:431–8. doi:10.3109/00016488209128931.

105. Bichler E, Spoendlin H, Rauchegger H. Degeneration of cochlear neurons after amikacin intoxication in the rat. Arch Otorhinolaryngol. 1983;237:201–8. doi:10.1007/BF00453725.

106. Alam SA, Robinson BK, Huang J, Green SH. Prosurvival and proapoptotic intracellular signaling in rat spiral ganglion neurons in vivo after the loss of hair cells. J Comp Neurol. 2007;503:832–52. doi:10.1002/cne.21430.

107. Leake PA, Hradek GT. Cochlear pathology of long term neomycin induced deafness in cats. Hear Res. 1988;33:11–33. doi:10.1016/0378-5955(88)90018-4.

108. Nadol Jr JB. Degeneration of cochlear neurons as seen in the spiral ganglion of man. Hear Res. 1990;49:141–54. doi:10.1016/0378-5955(90)90101-T.

109. Nadol Jr JB. Patterns of neural degeneration in the human cochlea and auditory nerve: implications for cochlear implantation. Otolaryngol Head Neck Surg. 1997;117:220–8. doi:10.1016/S0194-5998(97)70178-5.

110. Miller JM, Le Prell CG, Prieskorn DM, Wys NL, Altschuler RA. Delayed neurotrophin treatment following deafness rescues spiral ganglion cells from death and promotes regrowth of auditory nerve peripheral processes: effects of brain-derived neurotrophic factor and fibroblast growth factor. J Neurosci Res. 2007;85:1959–69. doi:10.1002/jnr.21320.

111. Leake PA, Hradek GT, Hetherington AM, Stakhovskaya O. Brain-derived neurotrophic factor promotes cochlear spiral ganglion cell survival and function in deafened, developing cats. J Comp Neurol. 2011;519:1526–45. doi:10.1002/cne.22582.

112. Landry TG, Wise AK, Fallon JB, Shepherd RK. Spiral ganglion neuron survival and function in the deafened cochlea following chronic neurotrophic treatment. Hear Res. 2011;282:303–13. doi:10.1016/j.heares.2011.06.007.

113. Glueckert R, Bitsche M, Miller JM, Zhu Y, Prieskorn DM, Altschuler RA, et al. Deafferentation-associated changes in afferent and efferent processes in the guinea pig cochlea and afferent regeneration with chronic intrascalar brain-derived neurotrophic factor and acidic fibroblast growth factor. J Comp Neurol. 2008;507:1602–21. doi:10.1002/cne.21619

114. Wise AK, Richardson R, Hardman J, Clark G, O'Leary S. Resprouting and survival of guinea pig cochlear neurons in response to the administration of the neurotrophins brain-derived neurotrophic factor and neurotrophin-3. J Comp Neurol. 2005;487:147–65. doi:10.1002/cne.20563.

115. Agterberg MJ, Versnel H, de Groot JC, Smoorenburg GF, Albers FW, Klis SF. Morphological changes in spiral ganglion cells after intracochlear application of brain-derived neurotrophic factor in deafened guinea pigs. Hear Res. 2008;244:25–34. doi:10.1016/j.heares.2008.07.004.
116. McGuinness SL, Shepherd RK. Exogenous BDNF rescues rat spiral ganglion neurons in vivo. Otol Neurotol. 2005;26:1064–72. doi:10.1097/01.mao.0000185063.20081.50.
117. Shibata SB, Cortez SR, Beyer LA, Wiler JA, Di Polo A, Pfingst BE, et al. Transgenic BDNF induces nerve fiber regrowth into the auditory epithelium in deaf cochleae. Exp Neurol. 2010;223:464–72. doi:10.1016/j.expneurol.2010.01.011.
118. Kinoshita M, Kikkawa YS, Sakamoto T, Kondo K, Ishihara K, Konno T, et al. Safety, reliability, and operability of cochlear implant electrode arrays coated with biocompatible polymer. Acta Otolaryngol. 2015;135:320–7. doi:10.3109/00016489.2014.990580.
119. Kondo K. Neurogenesis and Differentiation of the spiral ganglion neurons MB ENT (Japanese). 2008;93:17–22.
120. Kondo K. Regeneration of the spiral ganglion neurons. J Clin Exp Med (Japanese). 2008;226:981–5.

Chapter 5
Genetics of Inner Ear Malformation and Cochlear Nerve Deficiency

Nobuko Yamamoto, Ayako Kanno, and Tatsuo Matsunaga

Abstract Studies on genetics of inner ear malformation and cochlear nerve deficiency have been successful in several diseases. Here, we described the current knowledge about the genetics of representative diseases. Among nonsyndromic hearing losses, we reviewed DFNB4 which is caused by mutations in the *SLC26A4* and DFN3 which is caused by mutations in *POU3F4*. Among syndromic hearing losses, we reviewed Waardenburg syndrome, branchio-oto-renal (BOR) syndrome, CHARGE syndrome, Okihiro syndrome, and distal renal tubular acidosis. For chromosomal disorders, trisomy 21 (Down syndrome), trisomy 18, trisomy 13, and 22q11.2 deletion syndrome (DiGeorge syndrome) were reviewed. Although causative genes are identified for only a part of inner ear malformation and cochlear nerve deficiency at present, the situation is likely to change rapidly because of the development of next-generation sequencing technologies. With accumulation of genotype-phenotype information for these auditory disorders, explanation for the causes and mechanisms of hearing loss will become more widely available, planning of medical care will be more effective, and genetic counseling will get more precise.

Keywords Nonsyndromic hearing loss • Syndromic hearing loss • Chromosomal disorders • Genes • Next-generation sequencing

N. Yamamoto • T. Matsunaga (✉)
Division of Hearing and Balance Research, National Institute of Sensory Organs, National Tokyo Medical Center, 2-5-1 Higashigaoka, Meguro, Tokyo 152-8902, Japan

Department of Otolaryngology, National Tokyo Medical Center, 2-5-1 Higashigaoka, Meguro, Tokyo 152-8902, Japan
e-mail: matsunagatatsuo@kankakuki.go.jp

A. Kanno
Division of Hearing and Balance Research, National Institute of Sensory Organs, National Tokyo Medical Center, 2-5-1 Higashigaoka, Meguro, Tokyo 152-8902, Japan

Department of Otolaryngology, Inagi Municipal Hospital, 1171 Oomaru, Inagi, Tokyo 206-0801, Japan

© Springer Science+Business Media Singapore 2017
K. Kaga (ed.), *Cochlear Implantation in Children with Inner Ear Malformation and Cochlear Nerve Deficiency*, Modern Otology and Neurotology,
DOI 10.1007/978-981-10-1400-0_5

5.1   Introduction

Genetics is one of the important causes of inner ear malformation and cochlear nerve deficiency. Inner ear malformation has been classified into Mondini dysplasia (dysplasia of bony and membranous labyrinth), large vestibular aqueduct syndrome (LVA syndrome), and Scheibe dysplasia (cochleosaccular dysplasia) by a classic way [1]. Mondini dysplasia may be found as an isolated malformation or in association with other symptoms in certain syndromes such as Pendred syndrome, Klippel-Feil syndrome, and DiGeorge syndrome and in chromosomal anomalies. Both autosomal dominant and recessive inheritance have been reported for the isolated form of Mondini dysplasia [2, 3]. LVA syndrome is frequently associated with Mondini dysplasia and may be found in patients with autosomal recessive nonsyndromic hearing loss (DFNB4) or in association with syndromes such as Pendred syndrome, branchio-oto-renal syndrome (BOR syndrome), distal renal tubular acidosis, Waardenburg syndrome, CHARGE syndrome, and Down syndrome. Scheibe dysplasia may occur in isolation or as part of a syndrome including keratitis-ichthyosis-deafness syndrome and congenital rubella syndrome. Cochlear nerve deficiency is frequently associated with inner ear malformation, but it may be found in patients without inner ear malformation. Cochlear nerve deficiency has also been reported in several syndromes including CHARGE syndrome, VATER RAPADILINO syndrome, Möbius syndrome, and Okihiro syndrome [4].

Lately, a classification system based on varying stages of inner ear organogenesis was proposed [5], and, then, another classification system which was also relevant to the varying stages of inner ear organogenesis was proposed [6, 7] (Fig. 5.1). In these days, the classification by Sennaroglu is widely used for planning of cochlear implantation in patients with malformed cochlea. The genetic causes have been

Fig. 5.1 Classification system of inner ear malformation which was relevant to the varying stages of inner ear organogenesis

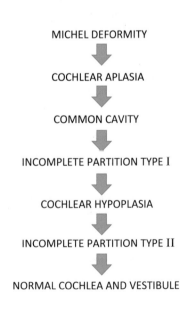

MICHEL DEFORMITY

COCHLEAR APLASIA

COMMON CAVITY

INCOMPLETE PARTITION TYPE I

COCHLEAR HYPOPLASIA

INCOMPLETE PARTITION TYPE II

NORMAL COCHLEA AND VESTIBULE

reported in a part of inner ear malformation classified by these systems, but they remain unknown in many others. In the following, we describe the current knowledge about the genetics of representative diseases presenting with inner ear malformation and cochlear nerve deficiency.

5.2 Nonsyndromic Hearing Loss

5.2.1 DFNB4/Pendred Syndrome

DFNB4 is characterized by a congenital severe-to-profound sensorineural hearing loss (SNHL). The hearing loss is described as bilateral, progressive, and fluctuant. There are episodes of sudden deterioration as well as vertigo. DFNB4 occurs as a recessively inherited disorder, genetically homogeneous, and is caused by biallelic mutations in the *SLC26A4* [8]. *SLC26A4* encodes a putative transmembrane protein designated pendrin, which functions as an anion transporter of chloride and iodide [9]. The *SLC26A4* consists of 21 exons and is located on chromosome 7 [10]. Studies in the mouse inner ear have shown that pendrin is expressed in epithelial cells that participate in regulating the composition of inner ear fluids and plays a role in development of the inner ear and in maintenance of normal homeostasis [11]. Radiological studies have shown that an enlargement of the endolymphatic sac and duct in association with a dilated vestibular aqueduct was found in the majority of cases [12], as well as a Mondini-type hypoplasia of the cochlea [13]. Mondini cochlea is a shortened cochlea, rudimentary modiolus, missing interscalar septum, and partial agenesis of the organ of Corti and cochlear neurons [14]. Association of symptoms such as goiter and a partial defect in iodide organification which develops in early puberty or adulthood is defined as Pendred syndrome.

5.2.2 DFN3

DFN3 is characterized by a mixed conductive-sensorineural moderate-to-profound hearing loss and occurrence of a perilymph gusher upon attempted fenestration of the stapes. DFN3 accounts for about half of all cases of X-linked hearing loss. The sensorineural hearing loss may be progressive, and the conductive component of hearing loss is characterized by an air-bone gap in the lower frequencies, often with preservation of the stapedial reflex [15]. The causative gene for DFN3 is *POU3F4* [16] which encodes a transcription factor POU3F4. POU3F4 belongs to the POU domain family and includes two functional domains, a POU-specific domain and a homeodomain [17]. *POU3F4* is expressed in the mesenchymal cells surrounding the otic vesicle during development [18]. The endocochlear potential was decreased in mutant mice [19], which is thought to be the cause of hearing loss. Radiological studies typically demonstrate dilatation of the internal auditory canal (IAC), often with deficiency of the bone between the IAC and the basal turn of the cochlea [15, 20]. Moreover, deficiency of the bone between the IAC and the vestibule, enlargement of the vestibular aqueduct, the absence of cochlear bony modioli, enlarged labyrinthine facial nerve canals, and dilated singular nerve canals [21] have been suggested. Sennaroglu et al. proposed a new classification for this type of inner ear malformation, namely, incomplete partition type III [7].

5.3 Syndromic Hearing Loss

5.3.1 Waardenburg Syndrome

Waardenburg syndrome was reported to occur in 1 in 42,000 of the population or 1.43 % of the congenitally deaf [22]. The characteristic features were (1) dystopia canthorum (lateral displacement of the medial canthi and lacrimal puncta), (2) broad nasal root, (3) confluence of the medial portions of the eyebrows, (4) partial or total heterochromia iridis, (5) circumscribed albinism of the frontal head hair (white forelock), and (6) sensorineural hearing loss (bilateral or unilateral). Waardenburg syndrome has been divided into four types, depending on the phenotype and presence of additional features. Types I and II are distinguished from each other by the presence of dystopia canthorum (type I) or by its absence (type II). Type III is characterized by the presence of limb defects and is also referred to as Klein-Waardenburg syndrome. Type IV accompanies Hirschsprung disease, which is known as the Shah-Waardenburg syndrome. Types I and II are more common. Waardenburg syndrome is genetically heterogeneous, with mutations reported in a number of different genes, which generally encode for transcription factors. These particular transcription factors appear to be critically involved in the differentiation, migration, and function of melanocytes. Melanocytes are widely distributed within the cochlea and vestibular sense organs. The types I and III are caused by mutations in the *PAX3* gene, which maps to 2q35. Inheritance is autosomal dominant [23]. The type II can be due to a mutation in the *MITF* gene, which maps to 3p14.1-p12.3, or in the *SNAI2* gene, which maps to 8q11 [24]. Inheritance is autosomal dominant in mutations involving *MITF* and autosomal recessive for *SNAI2*. The type IV can be caused by mutations in the *EDNRB* gene [25], the *EDN3* gene [26], or the *SOX10* gene [27]. The type IV may be either autosomal recessive or dominant in its inheritance. Recent reports indicated that the *EDNRB*, the *EDN3*, and the *SOX10* gene mutations could be involved in type II, although they were not a major cause of type II [28].

Recent reports have suggested that the frequency of hearing loss in type I is 58–75 % and in type II, 78–91 % [29–31]. The extents of loss and audiogram shapes are quite variable, ranging from no measurable clinical loss to severe congenital unilateral or bilateral sensorineural loss [30, 32]. Bilateral loss is more common. The hearing loss in type II has been found to be progressive in 70 % [32].

Abnormalities of the vestibular system are also common and may be seen in individuals who have normal hearing. Whereas the commonest pathological defect is of the Scheibe or cochleosaccular type, more major defects affecting the vestibular apparatus may occasionally be found.

5.3.2   BOR Syndrome

BOR syndrome is characterized by hearing loss, malformations of the external ear, branchial arch anomalies, and renal abnormalities. A mixed hearing loss is the most common type and the hearing loss is usually severe but can vary from mild to profound. Age of onset varies from early childhood to young adulthood. It is stable in majority of patients, although progressive hearing loss and fluctuant hearing loss have been described [33]. Malformations of the external ear include various types of abnormalities of the pinnae, stenosis of atresia of the external auditory canals, and the presence of helical or preauricular pits [34]. Mutations in the *EYA1* or *SIX1* have been identified to be the causative genes of BOR syndrome. *EYA1* is the most frequent causative gene which was first reported by Abdelhak et al. *EYA1* is located on chromosome 8q13.3 and acts as a protein phosphatase and transcriptional coactivator [35]. *SIX1* is another causative gene located on chromosome 14q23.1 [36]. *SIX1* interacts with *EYA1* in transcriptional regulation and involves in the development of the mammalian ear and kidney [37–39]. Radiological studies show a wide variety of middle ear and inner ear abnormalities including malformations or absence of the oval window, enlargement of the vestibular aqueduct, and Mondini anomalies [40].

5.3.3   CHARGE Syndrome

The CHARGE syndrome was described with the diagnosis based on patients having at least four of the following six abnormalities: (1) coloboma, (2) heart anomalies, (3) atresia choanae, (4) retarded physical and central nervous system growth, (5) genital hypoplasia, and (6) ear anomalies with hearing loss. The ear is almost always affected. Most CHARGE ears are short and wide. The most detailed study [41] reveals hearing loss in approximately 85 % of patients. Although several studies documented mixed hearing loss due to ossicular anomalies and/or middle ear effusion, many authors reported predominantly or exclusively sensorineural hearing loss [42]. The sensorineural component ranged from mild to severe or profound and was suspected congenital. The majority of patients had sloping sensorineural losses. Guyot et al. [43] pointed out a specific form of unusual dysplasia of the labyrinth characterized by severe dysplasia or agenesis of the pars superior (utricle and canals) and Mondini anomaly of the pars inferior (cochlea and saccule). However, there appear to be exceptions to this rule.

Most cases with the CHARGE syndrome are sporadic, but there is evidence of familial transmission supporting autosomal dominant and autosomal recessive inheritance. *CHD7* mutations occur in 32–64 % of patients with CHARGE syndrome features [44]. The most common mutations are nonsense and frameshift, but missense mutations can also occur. These various mutations cause haploinsufficiency of *CHD7*. In general, those with missense mutations tend to have milder and more variable phenotype than did those with truncating mutations [45]. The CHD7 protein appears to bind mostly to the DNA distal to transcriptional start sites of specific gene targets, enhancing their transcription either positively or negatively [46]. Abnormalities in the development, migration, or interaction of the cell of the neural crest may contribute to the pathogenesis of the CHARGE syndrome [47]. There has also been one report of a child with a clinical diagnosis of CHARGE syndrome who was found to have a mutation in semaphorin 3E (*SEMA3E*) [48].

5.3.4 Okihiro Syndrome

In 1977, Okihiro et al. [49] described a family of Duane syndrome (bilateral absence of adduction with widening on attempted abduction), most of whom had upper limb malformation and congenital severe sensorineural hearing loss. Inheritance is clearly autosomal dominant. Pathogenic mutations have been identified in the human *SALL4* gene at 20q13 in affected individuals [50]. Reporting nonsense and frameshift mutations in five of eight families studied, Kohlhase et al. [50] drew attention to the clinical overlap with Holt-Oram syndrome, acro-renal-ocular syndrome, and cases mistakenly diagnosed as representing thalidomide embryopathy.

5.3.5 Distal Renal Tubular Acidosis (DRTA)

DRTA is characterized by dehydration, growth impairment, metabolic acidosis with alkaline urine, and hearing loss. Mild-to-profound SNHL, mainly at higher frequencies, is seen in childhood. There are several reports with the progressive hearing loss [51, 52]. The inherence pattern of DRTA is autosomal recessive, and mutations in two genes, *ATP6V1B1* on chromosome 2p13 and *ATP6V0A4* on chromosome 7p33-34, are responsible [53, 54]. *ATP6V1B1* and *ATP6V0A4* code for subunits of vacuolar H^+-ATPase pump which serves to stabilize pH in both the kidney and inner ear [55]. Early SNHL occurs in most patients with *ATP6V1B1* mutations, whereas late-onset SNHL is seen with *ATP6V0A4* mutations [56]. High-resolution magnetic resonance imaging (MRI) performed in the patients demonstrated enlarged vestibular aqueducts, which can be unilateral or bilateral [55, 56].

5.4 Chromosomal Disorders Associated with Hearing Loss

5.4.1 Trisomy 21 (Down Syndrome)

Down syndrome, with an incidence of 1/600 live births, is the most common chromosome defect in humans. Ninety-five percent of Down syndrome is caused by an extra copy of a normal chromosome 21, such that the individual has a total of 47 chromosomes with three 21s (47,+21) in all cells. Two percent to four percent of cases are mosaic for the extra chromosome 21; that is, not all cells have trisomy 21. This can be the result of either meiotic or mitotic nondisjunction. In <5 % of Down syndrome cases, the additional 21 is caused by the presence of a chromosome rearrangement that results in the additional 21 being translocated to another chromosome. Most often, this occurs as a Robertsonian translocation, where the short arm of the 21 is translocated to the short arm of one of the other acrocentric chromosomes. These cases are significant in that the translocation can be inherited from a phenotypically normal parent, who is a balanced translocation carrier. Since 21 is the smallest chromosome with the fewest number of genes, the gene dosage imbalance resultant from the extra chromosome is one of the few autosomal trisomies tolerated during development, although only about 30 % of Down syndrome fetuses survive to the term [57].

The clinical manifestations are varied and include brachycephaly, upslanting palpebral fissures, epicanthic folds, short neck, flat nasal bridge, abnormalities of the pinnae, narrow palate, transverse palmar crease, mental retardation, congenital heart disease, short stature, duodenal atresia or stenosis, and cataracts [34]. The external ears tend to be small, apparently low set, and slightly posteriorly rotated. Temporal bones of Down syndrome patients show both middle and inner ear defects. Cochlear defects include Mondini dysplasia and overall hypoplasia in inner ear structures, including vestibular malformations and narrowing of the cochlear nerve canal [58]. Stapes malformations, residual mesenchyme obstructing the round window, and otitis media account for most middle ear structural abnormalities. Hearing loss is reported in over 80 % of children with Down syndrome [59]. Hearing loss can be conductive, sensorineural, or mixed.

5.4.2 Trisomy 18 (Edwards Syndrome)

The incidence is 1 in 5000 births. There is marked preponderance of females (3:1). Full trisomy 18 is the norm. A handful of mosaic cases have been reported [60]. Half of trisomy 18 newborns die within the first week; 90 % die within the first year of life [61]. Mosaicism for trisomy 18 may lead to partial expression of the phenotype, from mild to almost full expression. Among the constellations of abnormalities are hypoplasia of skeletal muscle; polyhydramnios; prominent occiput; narrow palpebral fissures; microstomia and micrognathia; microcephaly; clenched fist with the index finger overlapping the third and fourth fingers; shortened big toe; defects of the heart, lungs, and kidneys; hernias; cleft lip and/or palate; choanal atresia; slanting eyes; microphthalmia; low-set ears; and aural atresia [34]. Ears are low set, posteriorly rotated, and malformed and can have atresia of the external auditory canal. Temporal bone studies show abnormalities of the middle and inner ear, including failed ossification of the malleus, incus, and stapes, and retarded development of the cochlea [62]. It is likely that most babies with trisomy 18 are deaf or severely hearing impaired; however, audiometric analysis has not been reported.

5.4.3   Trisomy 13 (Patau Syndrome)

The incidence of trisomy 13 at birth is about 1 in 12,000. Babies born with trisomy 13 rarely survive more than a few days, and only 5 % survive to 6 months of age [57]. The majority of trisomy 13 cases are full free-lying trisomies, i.e., 47 chromosomes. Robertsonian translocation of a 13 onto another acrocentric chromosome has also been reported [63]. Among the anomalies are microcephaly and severe mental retardation, wide sagittal sutures and fontanels, gross anatomic defects of the brain, myelomeningocele, microphthalmia, iris colobomas, cleft lip and palate, antimongoloid slant eyes, simian palmar crease, polydactyly, rocker bottom feet, cardiac defects, low-set ears, and hearing loss [34]. Temporal bone studies show multiple abnormalities of the cochlea and vestibular systems, including semicircular canal and utricular, saccular, and macular anomalies; shortened cochlear length; widened cochlear aqueduct; and abnormalities of the modiolus and defects of the cochlear and vestibular nerves. Middle ear anomalies were also occasionally present [64]. Although hearing ability is often not evaluated because of the combined clinical and neurological impairments, one report noted at least two cases of documented hearing loss in mosaic trisomy 13 cases [63].

5.4.4   22q11.2 Deletion Syndrome (DiGeorge Syndrome)

The incidence of 22q11.2 deletion syndrome is 1 in 4000 [57]. DiGeorge syndrome is characterized by the agenesis of the thymus and parathyroid glands in association with other developmental anomalies of the third and fourth pharyngeal clefts, the cardiovascular and renal systems, and the craniofacial structures [34]. Eighty-five percent to Ninety percent of 22q11.2 deletion syndrome cases have a common deletion of 3 Mb at 22q11.2. Eight percent to ten percent of cases have a 1.5–2 Mb deletion at the same band [65]. The deletions are the result of chromosome 22-specific low-copy repeats that cause nonallelic homologous recombination. Studies in mice and humans have suggested that mutations in the TBX1 gene which maps to the center of the DiGeorge syndrome chromosomal region on 22q11.2 may be responsible for this phenotype [66]. Deletions at the second DiGeorge syndrome locus, 10p13, are larger and often seen on routine cytogenetics, but occur 50 times less frequently than the 22q11.2 deletions [67].

Patients with DiGeorge syndrome can have both external and inner ear defects. Auricular anomalies, one or more of which may be present in 80 % of cases, include small, low-set, or rotated ears; cupped or protruding ears; and helical anomalies [68]. More recent studies find 40 to 65 % of patients with hearing loss of greater than 25 dB in at least one ear [69, 70]; however, hearing deficits of more than 40 dB are relatively rare. The vast majority of hearing loss is conductive (70 to 90 %) and due to chronic otitis media. DiGeorge syndrome patients with a deletion at 10p13 compared to the classical 22q11.1 deletion appear to have a higher percentage of sensorineural hearing loss (41 % of patients). The hearing loss tends to be bilateral and progressive, ranging in a loss from 40 dB to profound loss [71]. Temporal bone studies note a variety of defects in some 22q11.2 deletion syndrome patients, including Mondini dysplasia, shortened cochlea, and defects of the outer and middle ear such as atresia of the external auditory canals and ossicular defects [70].

5.5 Perspective

Since the next-generation sequencing was introduced for the genetic analysis of hearing loss [72, 73], the discovery of novel deafness genes and genetic diagnosis of hearing loss have been greatly facilitated. Although causative genes are identified for only a part of inner ear malformation and cochlear nerve deficiency at present, the situation is likely to change rapidly. With accumulation of genotype-phenotype information for these auditory disorders, explanation for the causes and mechanisms of hearing loss will become more widely available, planning of medical care will be more effective, and genetic counseling will get more precise. Even without genetic testing, such information would contribute to physicians in understanding and predicting the causes and clinical characteristics of each type of the anomaly, which would benefit the medical intervention for patients who do not want genetic tests or prior to genetic tests.

References

1. Merchant SN. Anomalies of the inner ear. In: Merchant SN, Nadol JB, editors. Schuknecht's pathology of the ear. 3rd ed. Shelton: People's Medical Publishing House-USA; 2010. p. 262–77.
2. Chan KH, Eelkema EA, Furman JM, Kamerer DB. Familial sensorineural hearing loss: a correlative study of audiologic, radiographic, and vestibular findings. Ann Otol Rhinol Laryngol. 1991;100(8):620–5.
3. Griffith AJ, Telian SA, Downs C, Gorski JL, Gebarski SS, Lalwani AK, et al. Familial Mondini dysplasia. Laryngoscope. 1998;108(9):1368–73.

4. Bamiou DE, Worth S, Phelps P, Sirimanna T, Rajput K. Eighth nerve aplasia and hypoplasia in cochlear implant candidates: the clinical perspective. Otol Neurotol. 2001;22(4):492–6.
5. Jackler RK, Luxford WM, House WF. Congenital malformations of the inner ear: a classification based on embryogenesis. Laryngoscope. 1987;97(3 Pt 2 Suppl 40):2–14.
6. Sennaroglu L, Saatci I. A new classification for cochleovestibular malformations. Laryngoscope. 2002;112(12):2230–41. doi:10.1097/00005537-200212000-00019.
7. Sennaroglu L, Sarac S, Ergin T. Surgical results of cochlear implantation in malformed cochlea. Otol Neurotol. 2006;27(5):615–23. doi:10.1097/01.mao.0000224090.94882.b4.
8. Pryor SP, Madeo AC, Reynolds JC, Sarlis NJ, Arnos KS, Nance WE, et al. SLC26A4/PDS genotype-phenotype correlation in hearing loss with enlargement of the vestibular aqueduct (EVA): evidence that Pendred syndrome and non-syndromic EVA are distinct clinical and genetic entities. J Med Genet. 2005;42(2):159–65. doi:10.1136/jmg.2004.024208.
9. Scott DA, Wang R, Kreman TM, Sheffield VC, Karniski LP. The Pendred syndrome gene encodes a chloride-iodide transport protein. Nat Genet. 1999;21(4):440–3. doi:10.1038/7783.
10. Everett LA, Glaser B, Beck JC, Idol JR, Buchs A, Heyman M, et al. Pendred syndrome is caused by mutations in a putative sulphate transporter gene (PDS). Nat Genet. 1997;17(4):411–22. doi:10.1038/ng1297-411.
11. Royaux IE, Belyantseva IA, Wu T, Kachar B, Everett LA, Marcus DC, et al. Localization and functional studies of pendrin in the mouse inner ear provide insight about the etiology of deafness in pendred syndrome. J Assoc Res Otolaryngol. 2003;4(3):394–404.
12. Phelps PD, Coffey RA, Trembath RC, Luxon LM, Grossman AB, Britton KE, et al. Radiological malformations of the ear in Pendred syndrome. Clin Radiol. 1998;53(4):268–73.
13. Cremers CW, Admiraal RJ, Huygen PL, Bolder C, Everett LA, Joosten FB, et al. Progressive hearing loss, hypoplasia of the cochlea and widened vestibular aqueducts are very common features in Pendred's syndrome. Int J Pediatr Otorhinolaryngol. 1998;45(2):113–23.
14. Johnsen T, Jorgensen MB, Johnsen S. Mondini cochlea in Pendred's syndrome. A histological study. Acta Otolaryngol. 1986;102(3–4):239–47.
15. Cremers CW, Snik AF, Huygen PL, Joosten FB, Cremers FP. X-linked mixed deafness syndrome with congenital fixation of the stapedial footplate and perilymphatic gusher (DFN3). Adv Otorhinolaryngol. 2002;61:161–7.
16. de Kok YJ, van der Maarel SM, Bitner-Glindzicz M, Huber I, Monaco AP, Malcolm S, et al. Association between X-linked mixed deafness and mutations in the POU domain gene POU3F4. Science. 1995;267(5198):685–8.
17. Mathis JM, Simmons DM, He X, Swanson LW, Rosenfeld MG. Brain 4: a novel mammalian POU domain transcription factor exhibiting restricted brain-specific expression. EMBO J. 1992;11(7):2551–61.
18. Phippard D, Lu L, Lee D, Saunders JC, Crenshaw 3rd EB. Targeted mutagenesis of the POU-domain gene Brn4/Pou3f4 causes developmental defects in the inner ear. J Neurosci. 1999;19(14):5980–9.
19. Minowa O, Ikeda K, Sugitani Y, Oshima T, Nakai S, Katori Y, et al. Altered cochlear fibrocytes in a mouse model of DFN3 nonsyndromic deafness. Science. 1999;285(5432):1408–11.
20. Phelps PD, Reardon W, Pembrey M, Bellman S, Luxom L. X-linked deafness, stapes gushers and a distinctive defect of the inner ear. Neuroradiology. 1991;33(4):326–30.
21. Talbot JM, Wilson DF. Computed tomographic diagnosis of X-linked congenital mixed deafness, fixation of the stapedial footplate, and perilymphatic gusher. Am J Otol. 1994;15(2):177–82.
22. Waardenburg PJ. A new syndrome combining developmental anomalies of the eyelids, eyebrows and nose root with pigmentary defects of the iris and head hair and with congenital deafness. Am J Hum Genet. 1951;3(3):195–253.
23. Farrer LA, Grundfast KM, Amos J, Arnos KS, Asher Jr JH, Beighton P, et al. Waardenburg syndrome (WS) type I is caused by defects at multiple loci, one of which is near ALPP on chromosome 2: first report of the WS consortium. Am J Hum Genet. 1992;50(5):902–13.

24. Hughes AE, Newton VE, Liu XZ, Read AP. A gene for Waardenburg syndrome type 2 maps close to the human homologue of the microphthalmia gene at chromosome 3p12-p14.1. Nat Genet. 1994;7(4):509–12. doi:10.1038/ng0894-509.

25. Attie T, Till M, Pelet A, Amiel J, Edery P, Boutrand L, et al. Mutation of the endothelin-receptor B gene in Waardenburg-Hirschsprung disease. Hum Mol Genet. 1995;4(12):2407–9.

26. Edery P, Attie T, Amiel J, Pelet A, Eng C, Hofstra RM, et al. Mutation of the endothelin-3 gene in the Waardenburg-Hirschsprung disease (Shah-Waardenburg syndrome). Nat Genet. 1996;12(4):442–4. doi:10.1038/ng0496-442.

27. Pingault V, Bondurand N, Kuhlbrodt K, Goerich DE, Prehu MO, Puliti A, et al. SOX10 mutations in patients with Waardenburg-Hirschsprung disease. Nat Genet. 1998;18(2):171–3. doi:10.1038/ng0298-171.

28. Pingault V, Ente D, Dastot-Le Moal F, Goossens M, Marlin S, Bondurand N. Review and update of mutations causing Waardenburg syndrome. Hum Mutat. 2010;31(4):391–406. doi:10.1002/humu.21211.

29. Liu XZ, Newton VE, Read AP. Waardenburg syndrome type II: phenotypic findings and diagnostic criteria. Am J Med Genet. 1995;55(1):95–100. doi:10.1002/ajmg.1320550123.

30. Newton V. Hearing loss and Waardenburg's syndrome: implications for genetic counselling. J Laryngol Otol. 1990;104(2):97–103.

31. Oysu C, Oysu A, Aslan I, Tinaz M. Temporal bone imaging findings in Waardenburg's syndrome. Int J Pediatr Otorhinolaryngol. 2001;58(3):215–21.

32. Hildesheimer M, Maayan Z, Muchnik C, Rubinstein M, Goodman RM. Auditory and vestibular findings in Waardenburg's type II syndrome. J Laryngol Otol. 1989;103(12):1130–3.

33. Kemperman MH, Stinckens C, Kumar S, Huygen PL, Joosten FB, Cremers CW. Progressive fluctuant hearing loss, enlarged vestibular aqueduct, and cochlear hypoplasia in branchio-oto-renal syndrome. Otol Neurotol. 2001;22(5):637–43.

34. Merchant SN. Genetically determined and other developmental defects. In: Merchant SN, Nadol JB, editors. Schuknecht's pathology of the ear. 3rd ed. Shelton: People's Medical Publishing House-USA; 2010. p. 152–8, 191–215.

35. Abdelhak S, Kalatzis V, Heilig R, Compain S, Samson D, Vincent C, et al. A human homologue of the Drosophila eyes absent gene underlies branchio-oto-renal (BOR) syndrome and identifies a novel gene family. Nat Genet. 1997;15(2):157–64. doi:10.1038/ng0297-157.

36. Ruf RG, Xu PX, Silvius D, Otto EA, Beekmann F, Muerb UT, et al. SIX1 mutations cause branchio-oto-renal syndrome by disruption of EYA1-SIX1-DNA complexes. Proc Natl Acad Sci U S A. 2004;101(21):8090–5. doi:10.1073/pnas.0308475101.

37. Kalatzis V, Sahly I, El-Amraoui A, Petit C. Eya1 expression in the developing ear and kidney: towards the understanding of the pathogenesis of Branchio-Oto-Renal (BOR) syndrome. Dev Dyn. 1998;213(4):486–99. doi:10.1002/(SICI)1097-0177(199812)213:4<486::AID-AJA 13>3.0.CO;2-L.

38. Xu PX, Zheng W, Huang L, Maire P, Laclef C, Silvius D. Six1 is required for the early organogenesis of mammalian kidney. Development. 2003;130(14):3085–94.

39. Zheng W, Huang L, Wei ZB, Silvius D, Tang B, Xu PX. The role of Six1 in mammalian auditory system development. Development. 2003;130(17):3989–4000.

40. Ceruti S, Stinckens C, Cremers CW, Casselman JW. Temporal bone anomalies in the branchio-oto-renal syndrome: detailed computed tomographic and magnetic resonance imaging findings. Otol Neurotol. 2002;23(2):200–7.

41. Thelin JW, Mitchell JA, Hefner MA, Davenport SL. CHARGE syndrome. Part II. Hearing loss. Int J Pediatr Otorhinolaryngol. 1986;12(2):145–63.

42. Goldson E, Smith AC, Stewart JM. The CHARGE association. How well can they do? Am J Dis Child. 1986;140(9):918 21.

43. Guyot JP, Gacek RR, DiRaddo P. The temporal bone anomaly in CHARGE association. Arch Otolaryngol Head Neck Surg. 1987;113(3):321–4.

44. Bartels CF, Scacheri C, White L, Scacheri PC, Bale S. Mutations in the CHD7 gene: the experience of a commercial laboratory. Genet Test Mol Biomarkers. 2010;14(6):881–91. doi:10.1089/gtmb.2010.0101.
45. Bergman JE, Janssen N, Hoefsloot LH, Jongmans MC, Hofstra RM, van Ravenswaaij-Arts CM. CHD7 mutations and CHARGE syndrome: the clinical implications of an expanding phenotype. J Med Genet. 2011;48(5):334–42. doi:10.1136/jmg.2010.087106.
46. Schnetz MP, Handoko L, Akhtar-Zaidi B, Bartels CF, Pereira CF, Fisher AG, et al. CHD7 targets active gene enhancer elements to modulate ES cell-specific gene expression. PLoS Genet. 2010;6(7):e1001023. doi:10.1371/journal.pgen.1001023.
47. Siebert JR, Graham Jr JM, MacDonald C. Pathologic features of the CHARGE association: support for involvement of the neural crest. Teratology. 1985;31(3):331–6. doi:10.1002/tera.1420310303.
48. Lalani SR, Safiullah AM, Molinari LM, Fernbach SD, Martin DM, Belmont JW. SEMA3E mutation in a patient with CHARGE syndrome. J Med Genet. 2004;41(7):e94.
49. Okihiro MM, Tasaki T, Nakano KK, Bennett BK. Duane syndrome and congenital upper-limb anomalies. A familial occurrence. Arch Neurol. 1977;34(3):174–9.
50. Kohlhase J, Schubert L, Liebers M, Rauch A, Becker K, Mohammed SN, et al. Mutations at the SALL4 locus on chromosome 20 result in a range of clinically overlapping phenotypes, including Okihiro syndrome, Holt-Oram syndrome, acro-renal-ocular syndrome, and patients previously reported to represent thalidomide embryopathy. J Med Genet. 2003;40(7):473–8.
51. Bourke E, Delaney VB, Mosawi M, Reavey P, Weston M. Renal tubular acidosis and osteopetrosis in siblings. Nephron. 1981;28(6):268–72.
52. Brown MT, Cunningham MJ, Ingelfinger JR, Becker AN. Progressive sensorineural hearing loss in association with distal renal tubular acidosis. Arch Otolaryngol Head Neck Surg. 1993;119(4):458–60.
53. Karet FE, Finberg KE, Nelson RD, Nayir A, Mocan H, Sanjad SA, et al. Mutations in the gene encoding B1 subunit of H+-ATPase cause renal tubular acidosis with sensorineural deafness. Nat Genet. 1999;21(1):84–90. doi:10.1038/5022.
54. Karet FE, Finberg KE, Nayir A, Bakkaloglu A, Ozen S, Hulton SA, et al. Localization of a gene for autosomal recessive distal renal tubular acidosis with normal hearing (rdRTA2) to 7q33-34. Am J Hum Genet. 1999;65(6):1656–65. doi:10.1086/302679.
55. Andreucci E, Bianchi B, Carboni I, Lavoratti G, Mortilla M, Fonda C, et al. Inner ear abnormalities in four patients with dRTA and SNHL: clinical and genetic heterogeneity. Pediatr Nephrol. 2009;24(11):2147–53. doi:10.1007/s00467-009-1261-3.
56. Stover EH, Borthwick KJ, Bavalia C, Eady N, Fritz DM, Rungroj N, et al. Novel ATP6V1B1 and ATP6V0A4 mutations in autosomal recessive distal renal tubular acidosis with new evidence for hearing loss. J Med Genet. 2002;39(11):796–803.
57. Morton CC, Giersch ABS. Genetic hearing loss associated with chromosome disorders. In: Toriello HV, Smith SD, editors. Hereditary hearing loss and its syndromes. 3rd ed. New York: Oxford University Press; 2013. p. 701–14.
58. Blaser S, Propst EJ, Martin D, Feigenbaum A, James AL, Shannon P, et al. Inner ear dysplasia is common in children with Down syndrome (trisomy 21). Laryngoscope. 2006;116(12):2113–9. doi:10.1097/01.mlg.0000245034.77640.4f.
59. Dahle AJ, McCollister FP. Hearing and otologic disorders in children with Down syndrome. Am J Ment Defic. 1986;90(6):636–42.
60. Schubert R, Eggermann T, Hofstaetter C, von Netzer B, Knopfle G, Schwanitz G. Clinical, cytogenetic, and molecular findings in 45, X/47, XX,+18 mosaicism: clinical report and review of the literature. Am J Med Genet. 2002;110(3):278–82. doi:10.1002/ajmg.10442.
61. Weber WW, Mamunes P, Day R, Miller P. Trisomy 17–18(E): studies in long-term survival with report of two autopsied cases. Pediatrics. 1964;34:533–41.
62. Chrobok V, Simakova E. Temporal bone findings in trisomy 18 and 21 syndromes. Eur Arch Otorhinolaryngol. 1997;254(1):15–8.

63. Delatycki M, Gardner RJ. Three cases of trisomy 13 mosaicism and a review of the literature. Clin Genet. 1997;51(6):403–7.
64. Fukushima H, Schachern PA, Cureoglu S, Paparella MM. Temporal bone study of trisomy 13 syndrome. Laryngoscope. 2008;118(3):506–7. doi:10.1097/MLG.0b013e31815b2176.
65. Emanuel BS, Shaikh TH. Segmental duplications: an 'expanding' role in genomic instability and disease. Nat Rev Genet. 2001;2(10):791–800. doi:10.1038/35093500.
66. Jerome LA, Papaioannou VE. DiGeorge syndrome phenotype in mice mutant for the T-box gene, Tbx1. Nat Genet. 2001;27(3):286–91. doi:10.1038/85845.
67. Berend SA, Spikes AS, Kashork CD, Wu JM, Daw SC, Scambler PJ, et al. Dual-probe fluorescence in situ hybridization assay for detecting deletions associated with VCFS/DiGeorge syndrome I and DiGeorge syndrome II loci. Am J Med Genet. 2000;91(4):313–7.
68. Ford LC, Sulprizio SL, Rasgon BM. Otolaryngological manifestations of velocardiofacial syndrome: a retrospective review of 35 patients. Laryngoscope. 2000;110(3 Pt 1):362–7. doi:10.1097/00005537-200003000-00006.
69. Reyes MR, LeBlanc EM, Bassila MK. Hearing loss and otitis media in velo-cardio-facial syndrome. Int J Pediatr Otorhinolaryngol. 1999;47(3):227–33.
70. Shprintzen RJ. Velocardiofacial syndrome. Otolaryngol Clin North Am. 2000;33(6):1217–40, vi.
71. Van Esch H, Groenen P, Fryns JP, Van de Ven W, Devriendt K. The phenotypic spectrum of the 10p deletion syndrome versus the classical DiGeorge syndrome. Genet Couns. 1999;10(1):59–65.
72. Shearer AE, DeLuca AP, Hildebrand MS, Taylor KR, Gurrola 2nd J, Scherer S, et al. Comprehensive genetic testing for hereditary hearing loss using massively parallel sequencing. Proc Natl Acad Sci U S A. 2010;107(49):21104–9. doi:10.1073/pnas.1012989107.
73. Walsh T, Shahin H, Elkan-Miller T, Lee MK, Thornton AM, Roeb W, et al. Whole exome sequencing and homozygosity mapping identify mutation in the cell polarity protein GPSM2 as the cause of nonsyndromic hearing loss DFNB82. Am J Hum Genet. 2010;87(1):90–4. doi:10.1016/j.ajhg.2010.05.010.

Chapter 6
Classification of Inner Ear Malformations

Levent Sennaroglu and Münir Demir Bajin

Abstract Morphologically congenital sensorineural hearing loss (SNHL) can be investigated under two categories. Majority of the congenital hearing loss (80 %) are membranous malformations. Here the pathology involves inner ear hair cells. There is no gross bony abnormality and, therefore, in these cases, high-resolution computerized tomography (HRCT) and magnetic resonance imaging (MRI) of the temporal bone revealed normal findings. The remaining 20 % have various malformations involving the bony labyrinth and, therefore, can be radiologically demonstrated by CT and MRI. The latter group involves surgical challenges as well as problems in decision-making. Some cases may be managed by hearing aid; some need cochlear implantation, while some cases are candidates for an auditory brainstem implantation. During cochlear implantation, there may be facial nerve abnormalities, cerebrospinal fluid leakage, electrode misplacement, or difficulty in finding the cochlea itself. During the surgery for inner ear malformations, the surgeon must be ready to modify the surgical approach or choose special electrodes for surgery.

Keywords Inner ear malformations • Cochleovestibular anomalies • Classification • Surgery

6.1 Introduction

Inner ear malformations (IEM) represent approximately 20 % of congenital hearing loss cases based on radiology [1]. The majority of these patients have bilateral severe to profound hearing loss and are candidates for cochlear implantation. Those cases with severe malformations may require special surgical approaches for implant placement. Decision-making between cochlear implantation (CI) and auditory brainstem implantation (ABI) may also be challenging in some cases of IEMs.

According to present literature [2–4], IEMs are classified into eight distinct groups.

L. Sennaroglu (✉) • M.D. Bajin
Department of Otolaryngology, Medical Faculty, Hacettepe University,
Sıhhiye 06100, Ankara, Turkey
e-mail: lsennaroglu@gmail.com

© Springer Science+Business Media Singapore 2017
K. Kaga (ed.), *Cochlear Implantation in Children with Inner Ear Malformation
and Cochlear Nerve Deficiency*, Modern Otology and Neurotology,
DOI 10.1007/978-981-10-1400-0_6

61

6.1.1 Complete Labyrinthine Aplasia (CLA, Michel Deformity)

6.1.1.1 Definition and Radiology

Labyrinthine aplasia is the absence of the cochlea, vestibule, semicircular canals, and vestibular and cochlear aqueducts (Figs. 6.1a, 6.1b and 6.1c). The petrous bone may be hypoplastic, whereas the otic capsule may be hypoplastic or aplastic [5]. In the majority of patients, the internal auditory canal (IAC) consists only of the facial canal and the labyrinthine; tympanic and mastoid segments of the facial nerve can be followed in the temporal bone. In some patients, however, it may not be possible to observe the facial canal in the temporal bone in spite of normal facial functions. Ossicles are usually present in the middle ear.

According to radiological findings [4], three different groups of CLA are present:

CLA with hypoplastic or aplastic petrous bone
In these cases CLA is accompanied by hypoplasia or aplasia of the petrous bone.
    The middle ear may be adjacent to the posterior fossa (Fig. 6.1a).
CLA without otic capsule
In this group of CLA, formation of the petrous bone is normal, but the otic capsule is hypoplastic or aplastic. According to Donaldson [6], the endosteum receives its vascular supply from the IAC, and the enchondral and outer periosteal layers get their vascular supply from the middle ear mucosa. This may be due to the abnormal vascular supply from the IAC and middle ear, resulting in the absence of all three layers of the otic capsule (Fig. 6.1b).

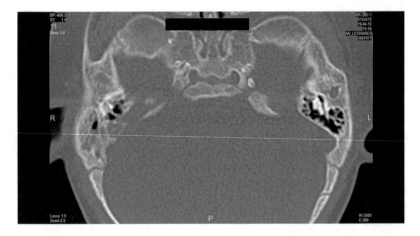

Fig. 6.1a Complete labyrinthine aplasia with hypoplastic petrous bone

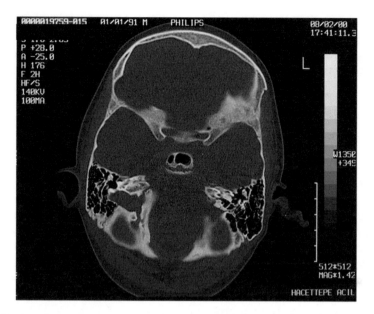

Fig. 6.1b Complete labyrinthine aplasia without otic capsule

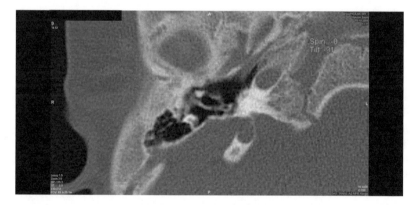

Fig. 6.1c Complete labyrinthine aplasia with otic capsule

CLA with otic capsule

Formation of the petrous bone and the otic capsule is normal. It can be speculated that vascular supply from the middle ear is normal as the otic capsule normally develops. The facial nerve canal can be seen (Fig. 6.1c). Only in this group of CLA with otic capsule development, the facial canal is in its normal location. This shows that otic capsule formation is essential for the facial canal to obtain its normal position.

6.1.1.2 Audiological Findings

Audiological examination reveals either no response at all or profound sensorineural hearing loss (SNHL) at 125, 250 and 500 Hz at the upper limits of the audiometer which may be due to vibrotactile sensations.

6.1.1.3 Management

It is not possible to perform cochlear implant (CI) surgery in these children as there is no inner ear development. Auditory brainstem implantation (ABI) is thus the only surgical option for hearing habilitation. Although translabyrinthine, retrosigmoid, and retrolabyrinthine approaches can be used for ABI surgery, the retrosigmoid approach is preferred in children [7]: the temporal bone is much smaller in children of 2–3 years of age when compared to that of an adult. As a result, the translabyrinthine approach provides a much more limited surgical exposure than the retrosigmoid approach. In addition, in translabyrinthine approach drilling, the temporal bone to expose the brainstem requires longer surgical times compared to retrosigmoid craniotomy. Therefore, retrosigmoid approach is favored for ABI surgery in children.

6.1.2 Rudimentary Otocyst

6.1.2.1 Definition and Radiology

A rudimentary otocyst consists of incomplete millimetric representations of the otic capsule (round or ovoid in shape) without an IAC (Fig. 6.2). Sometimes parts of the semicircular canals may accompany rudimentary otocyst. This pathology represents an anomaly between a Michel deformity and common cavity. In Michel deformity, there is no inner ear development, while in common cavity (CC), there is an ovoid or round cystic space instead of a separate cochlea and vestibule. The CC communicates with the brainstem via the nerves in the IAC. The rudimentary otocyst is a few millimeters in size without the formation of an IAC.

The inner ear is in the form of an otocyst (otic vesicle) between the third and fourth week [4]. The insult probably occurs at the beginning of the formation of the otocyst and results in rudimentary otocyst deformity.

6.1.2.2 Management

The fact that there is no connection between the otocyst and the brainstem is a contraindication to CI surgery. As a result, these patients are candidates for ABI.

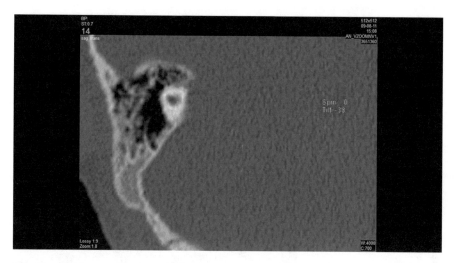

Fig. 6.2 Rudimentary otocyst

6.1.3   Cochlear Aplasia

6.1.3.1   Definition and Radiology

Cochlear aplasia is the absence of the cochlea. The accompanying vestibular system may be normal (Fig. 6.3a) or enlarged (Fig. 6.3b) [1]. The labyrinthine segment of the facial nerve is anteriorly displaced and occupies the normal location of the cochlea. Cochlear aplasia with a dilated vestibule (CADV) must be differentiated from common cavity (CC). If the cochleovestibular nerve (CVN) is present, cochlear implantation can be done in CC. However, CI surgery should not be done in CADV. In some patients, it may be very difficult to distinguish between these entities.

Cochlear aplasia with normal labyrinth is almost always symmetrical. The fact that similar findings are present in different patients suggests genetic etiology. In CADV, however, asymmetric development is present; pathology may be genetic or environmental. Otic capsule development is always normal.

After the development of the otic vesicle at the end of the fourth week, the membranous labyrinth develops in three areas: the cochlea, the vestibule, and the endolymphatic duct [4]. Cochlear aplasia is the absence of the cochlear duct, where vestibular and endolymphatic structures may develop normally. The time of the insult must be around the fifth week.

Fig. 6.3a Cochlear aplasia
with normal vestibular
system

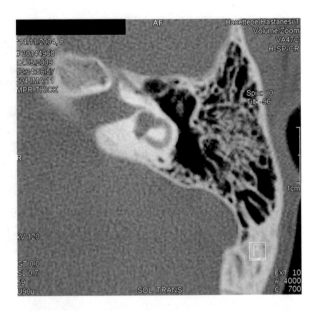

Fig. 6.3b Cochlear aplasia
with dilated vestibular
system

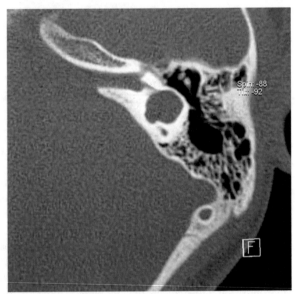

6.1.3.2 Audiological Findings

Typically, these patient will have no response at all or profound hearing loss at low frequencies. Collectively, these findings in complete labyrinthine aplasia, otocyst deformity, and cochlear aplasia demonstrate that profound hearing loss at low frequencies is purely a vibrotactile response and should not be interpreted as hearing in CI candidates with other pathologies.

6.1.3.3 Management

As there is no inner ear development, ABI is the only feasible surgical option to provide hearing in children with cochlear aplasia.

6.1.4 *Common Cavity*

6.1.4.1 Definition and Radiology

A common cavity is defined as a single chamber, ovoid or round in shape, representing the cochlea and vestibule (Fig. 6.4). Theoretically, this structure has cochlear and vestibular neural structures. There may be accompanying semicircular canals (SCC) or their rudimentary parts. The IAC usually enters the cavity at its center. Cases with vestibular dilatation are occasionally termed as "vestibular common cavity"; however, this is not a correct term.

Common cavity (CC) should be differentiated from cochlear aplasia with vestibular dilatation (CAVD) [1]. *Cochlear aplasia with vestibular dilatation* (CAVD) (Fig. 6.3b) usually has a vestibule and semicircular canals at their usual location at the posterolateral part of the IAC fundus. The external outline resembles the normal labyrinth. The vestibule is at its expected location. The accompanying SCCs may be enlarged or normal. A *common cavity* (CC) (Fig. 6.4), on the other hand, is an ovoid or round structure. SCCs or their rudimentary parts may accompany a common cavity. The IAC usually enters the cavity at its center. The location of a CC may be anterior or posterior to the normal location of the labyrinth. It is very important to

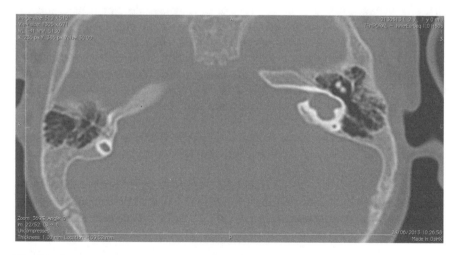

Fig. 6.4 Common cavity

differentiate these malformations from each other, because cochlear implantation in a CC may result in acoustic stimulation, whereas in CAVD, no functional stimulation will occur with CI. In spite of these factors, it may sometimes be difficult to differentiate between the two malformations.

CC contains cochlear and vestibular neural elements. This represents development arrest before there is a clear differentiation into the cochlea and vestibule: it is in between rudimentary otocyst and cochlear aplasia and usually occurs around the fourth to fifth week [4].

At the time of insult, the CC is only millimetric in size, as a developed otocyst. The CC may have small or large dimensions: usually, a CC with a diameter of 1–3 cm is encountered. This shows that its capacity to differentiate into the cochlea and vestibule may terminate, but it can still enlarge; so a CC larger than an initial otocyst may be encountered. IAC may be normal or narrow in a large CC. It appears that there is no relationship of the size of the IAC (length and width) and the size of the CC.

6.1.4.2 Audiological Findings

These patients can have detectable hearing thresholds only at low frequencies and at the maximum limits of the audiometer.

6.1.4.3 Management

Cochleovestibular nerve (CVN) should be demonstrated with high-resolution 3-tesla MRI before discussing management options with the family. At the present time, there is no test to determine the amount of cochlear fibers in the CVN [7]. If a behavioral audiometric response or language development is present with hearing aid use, it can be assumed that a meaningful population of cochlear fibers exists and the patient may benefit from a CI. The surgical approach is via a transmastoid labyrinthotomy as described by McElveen [8] with a straight (non-modiolar-hugging) electrode. This will have a position on the periphery of the CC with better contact with the neural tissue. A pre-curved electrode will have the contacts located medially and may not stimulate the periphery of the CC efficiently.

If the CVN cannot be demonstrated with MRI or there is a very narrow or long IAC, where the presence of cochlear fibers is questionable, an ABI may be a more appropriate option from the outset.

As the postoperative hearing cannot be accurately predicted before CI surgery, it is advisable to counsel the family that contralateral ABI may be necessary in case of limited language development with CI. This decision should be done as early as possible.

6.1.5   Hypoplasia and Incomplete Partitions

In these groups of malformations, there is a clear differentiation into a cochlea and vestibule.

6.1.5.1   Incomplete Partition of the Cochlea: Definition and Radiology

Incomplete partition anomalies represent a group of cochlear malformations with normal external dimensions and various internal architecture defects. Incomplete partitions constitute 41 % of inner ear malformations in the database of Hacettepe University Department of Otolaryngology. There are three different types of incomplete partition groups according to the defect in the modiolus and the interscalar septa.

6.1.5.2   Types of Incomplete Partition Groups

Incomplete Partition Type I (IP-I)

This type was termed as "cystic cochleovestibular malformation" in 2002 by Sennaroglu and Saatci [9]. These represent approximately 20 % of inner ear malformations. In this group, the cochlea lacks the entire modiolus and interscalar septa (Fig. 6.5a), giving the appearance of an empty cystic structure. IP-I cochlea has external dimensions (height and length) similar to normal cases [10]. It is accompanied by an enlarged, dilated vestibule (Fig. 6.5b). Vestibular aqueduct enlargement

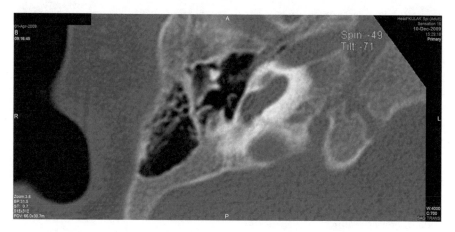

Fig. 6.5a   Incomplete partition type I without modiolus and interscalar septa

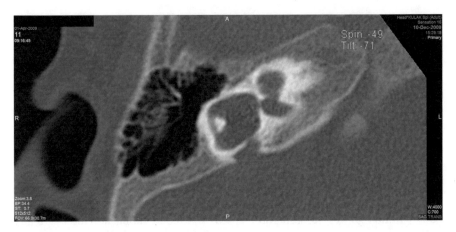

Fig. 6.5b Incomplete partition type I, with grossly dilated vestibule

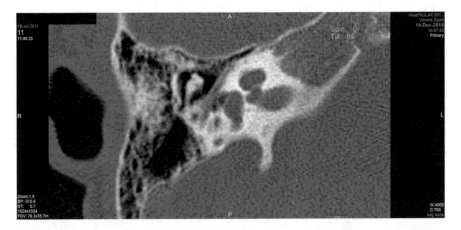

Fig. 6.5c *Incomplete partition type II* with defective modiolus, minimally dilated vestibule, and a large vestibular aqueduct

is very rare. There may be a defect between the IAC and the cochlea due to developmental abnormality of the cochlear aperture and the absence of the modiolus (Fig. 6.5c), and CSF may completely fill the cochlea. The cochlea is located in its usual location in the anterolateral part of the fundus of the IAC.

Recent histopathology study suggests that IP-I may be due to endosteal development abnormality as a result of defective vascular supply coming from the IAC [4].

Audiological Findings

The majority of IP-I patients have severe to profound SNHL. They are almost always candidates for CI.

During CI surgery gusher is very common which necessitates special precautions. Facial nerve abnormalities can also be seen as a result of abnormal development of the labyrinth. This may necessitate modification of the surgical approach.

As it is possible to have CN aplasia in IP-I, some patients may not be a candidate for CI surgery. Therefore, an ABI is indicated in IP-I patients with aplastic CN. Four patients with IP-I and an aplastic CN have received ABI in our department.

Recurrent meningitis can occur in IP-I patients even prior to their CI surgery or in their nonoperated ear. High CSF pressure filling the cochlea disrupts an often thin stapes footplate, leading to a CSF fistula at the oval window and meningitis. Several cases of this have been reported in the literature [11–14]. Spontaneous CSF fistula and recurrent meningitis can be seen although less frequently in cochlear hypoplasia type II. This is because both IP-I and CH-II have endosteal developmental anomaly leading to defective footplate development. If CSF fills the cochlea with high pressure, it may lead to a fistula. If the cochleostomy is not properly sealed, this may also lead to a CSF fistula with recurrent meningitis. It is interesting to note that IP-III cases almost always have a high-volume CSF gusher during CI surgery, but meningitis is very rarely reported in these patients [11, 14]. This is most likely due to the fact that the stapes footplate is normally developed because in IP-III pathology is in the outer two layers of the otic capsule and endosteum is normal. Therefore, a defect in the footplate is very unlikely.

All patients with IP-I and recurrent meningitis who have normal tympanic membranes but fluid filling the middle ear and mastoid should have an exploration of the middle ear with special attention to the stapes footplate.

Incomplete Partition Type II (IP-II)

In IP-II, the apical part of the modiolus is defective (Fig. 6.5d). This anomaly was originally described by Carlo Mondini and together with a minimally dilated vestibule and a large vestibular aqueduct (LVA) (Fig. 6.5d) constitutes the triad of the *Mondini deformity*. It is very important to use this particular name only if the above mentioned triad of malformations is present [1, 9, 11, 15]. The apical part of the modiolus and the corresponding interscalar septa are defective. This gives the apex of the cochlea a cystic appearance due to the confluence of middle and apical turns. The external dimensions of the cochlea (height and diameter) are similar to that seen in normal cases [10]. Therefore, it is not correct to define this anomaly as a cochlea with 1.5 turns [10]. This description should only be used for cochlear hypoplasia.

The recent study on histopathology demonstrated that modiolar defects may be due to high CSF pressure transmission into the inner ear as a result of LVA [4]. An enlarged endolymphatic sac and duct appears to be the only genetic abnormality that is causing the other abnormalities allowing high CSF pressure to be transmitted into the inner ear. This results in a mild dilatation in the walls of the vestibule.

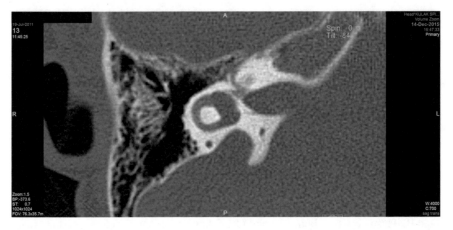

Fig. 6.5d Incomplete partition type II with defective modiolus, minimally dilated vestibule, and a large vestibular aqueduct

However, no hydropic changes were observed in the endolymphatic space. Depending on the severity and timing of the insult, the pathology may stay at this stage and cause LVA only, or with the transmission of CSF pressure into the cochlea, it may cause a spectrum of anomalies ranging from scala vestibuli dilatation and scala communis, superior (cystic apex) to partial, subtotal, and in some cases complete modiolar defects. The high pressure in the SV causes bulging of the ISS upward. This is a constant finding in all cases, showing that cochlear pathology may be the result of high pressure in the SV and that it happened during the developmental phase, otherwise high pressure would have caused fracture of the osseous spiral lamina. If there is higher pressure, it is natural to expect more destruction at the upper and, possibly, the lower part of the modiolus. This is the reason for the CSF oozing and gusher sometimes observed during CI surgery.

Audiological Findings

These patients do not have a characteristic hearing level, as their audiometric threshold testing varies from normal to profound. The hearing loss can be symmetric or asymmetric, but it is usually progressive. It is also possible to have sudden SNHL. In addition, there is an air-bone gap particularly present at low frequencies. Tympanometry is normal in the absence of otitis media and acoustic reflexes are generally present. Air-bone gap in these children is likely to be due to a "third-window" effect from the LVA and can resemble the audiometric findings in superior canal dehiscence syndrome.

Management

At a young age, these patients may have near normal hearing and usually do not require amplification initially. With progressive hearing loss, they become candidates for hearing aid. Usually the progression in hearing loss continues, ultimately

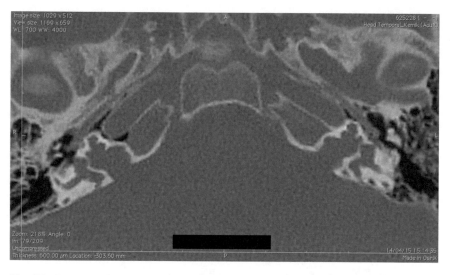

Fig. 6.5e Incomplete partition type III with interscalar septa but absent modiolus

creating a need for CI at some point in the future. High-pulsating CSF pressure may be responsible for the progression of hearing loss. A role for head trauma has been suggested, and these patients are advised to avoid trauma by wearing helmets when playing sports and avoiding contact sports completely.

During surgery, a facial recess approach was successfully used in all 67 patients who underwent CI surgery at Hacettepe University. As the cochlea and labyrinth have normal dimensions, facial nerve abnormality is very rare, and standard approach can be used in all patients.

Out of 67 patients operated on in our department, 32 patients had no CSF leakage, 29 patients had CSF oozing, and 6 patients had gusher. Even though there was no CSF leakage, all patients demonstrated strong pulsation at the time of cochleostomy. This finding may be used to explain the progressive nature of the hearing loss.

Gusher is more common in IP-I or IP-III, but it may occur in IP-II as well. This observation indicates the presence of a modiolar defect. An LVA cannot explain CSF leakage. The cochleostomy should be closed completely to avoid the risk of recurrent meningitis. As the basal part of the modiolus is normal, all kinds of electrodes (modiolar hugging, straight) can be used. Because of the risk of CSF leakage and sometimes severe gusher, electrodes with cork-type stopper may be advantageous. The surgeon must be prepared to use the measures to manage the CSF gusher.

Incomplete Partition Type III (IP-III)

The cochlea in IP-III has interscalar septa, but the modiolus is completely absent (Fig. 6.5e). IP-III cochlear malformation is the type of anomaly present in X-linked deafness, which was described by Nance et al. [16] for the first time in 1971. Phelps et al. [17] described the HRCT findings associated with this condition for the first time, and this characteristic deformity was included under the category of incomplete partition deformities for the first time by Sennaroglu et al. in 2006 [18].

This anomaly is the rarest form of incomplete partition cases. IP-III constitutes 2% of the IEMs in the database in Hacettepe University Department of Otolaryngology.

In an IP-III cochlea otic capsule around the membranous labyrinth is thinner when compared to that in a normal cochlea. HRCT demonstrates that in IP-III, the otic capsule around the cochlea is thin and follows the outline of the membranous labyrinth as if it is formed by a thick endosteal layer. Instead of the usual three layers, probably the second and third layers are either absent or very thin. The innermost endosteal layer appears to be thickened without enchondral and outer periosteal layers.

Radiology

Phelps et al. [17] reported that there is a bulbous IAC, incomplete separation of the coils of the cochlea from the IAC, and widened first and second parts of the intratemporal facial nerve canal with a less acute angle between them. Talbot and Wilson [19] later added that the modiolus is absent and there is a more medial origin of the vestibular aqueduct with varying degrees of dilatation.

In addition, Sennaroglu et al. [20] reported that in this deformity, the interscalar septa are present, but the modiolus is completely absent (Fig. 6.5e). The cochlea is located directly at the lateral end of the internal auditory canal instead of its usual anterolateral position. This gives the cochlea a characteristic appearance. From an earlier study, the external dimensions of the cochlea (height and diameter) were found to be similar to the normal cochlea [18]; therefore, it is appropriate to include IP-III under the incomplete partition anomalies. In addition, the labyrinthine segment of the facial nerve is located almost above the cochlea [21]. The labyrinthine segment of the facial nerve is the most superior structure in the temporal bone. The thin otic capsule around the cochlea and labyrinth, consisting of only thick endosteal layer, may be responsible for this. The tympanic and mastoid segments appear to be in normal position.

Audiological Findings

In IP-III there may be mixed-type HL or profound SNHL. Conductive component may be due to thin otic capsule. Stapes surgery should be avoided in this group. It may lead to gusher and further SNHL. They have excellent cochlear nerves. Therefore, ABI is not indicated in this group of incomplete partitions.

Management

Mixed hearing loss gives the impression of stapedial fixation. Stapedotomy results in severe gusher and further SNHL and, thus, should be avoided. Patients with severe HL are candidates for CI.

Because of the absent modiolus in IP-III, two serious problems may occur during CI surgery:

Gusher: Severe gusher always occurs due to the large defect between the cochlea and the IAC. If it is not properly sealed, the postoperative CSF leakage may lead to recurrent meningitis.

Electrode misplacement into the IAC: Because of the defective modiolus, electrodes with complete rings or contact surface on both sides may provide better stimulation. Modiolar-hugging electrodes have a tendency to go toward the center of the cochlea. As there is no modiolus in IP-III, this may result in misplacement into the IAC. The probability of the longer electrodes entering the IAC is more than the shorter electrodes. Therefore, an electrode with full rings or contact surfaces on both sides that will make only one turn around the cochlea appears to be sufficient.

If a modiolar-hugging electrode is used and postoperative x-ray demonstrates that the electrode is inside of the IAC, the facial and cochlear nerves may be damaged during electrode removal. Thus, straight electrodes that are 25 mm in length and provide one full turn around the cochlea are preferable.

Position of the electrode should be checked by an intraoperative x-ray. If the electrode is discovered to be in the IAC, it should be repositioned during surgery.

As mentioned above, spontaneous CSF leakage through the oval window is more frequently seen and reported in IP-I, even though both IP-I and IP-III are associated with high-volume CSF leakage on cochleostomy. This is most probably due to footplate defect as a result of endosteal developmental anomaly in IP-I. In IP-III endosteum is normally developed with thinner otic capsule due to defective outer layers. Therefore, spontaneous CSF leakage is very rare in IP-III.

6.1.6   Hypoplasia and Incomplete Partitions

In these groups of malformations, there is a clear differentiation between a cochlea and vestibule.

6.1.6.1   Cochlear Hypoplasia: Radiology and Definition

In this deformity, there is clear differentiation between the cochlea and vestibule. Cochlear hypoplasia represents a group of cochlear malformations with external dimensions less than those of a normal cochlea with various internal architecture deformities. In smaller cochlea, it is usually difficult to count the number of turns with CT and/or MRI. But the definition "cochlea with 1.5 turns" should be used for hypoplasia (particularly type III), rather than for IP-II cochlea. Four different types of cochlear hypoplasia have been defined.

6.1.6.2 Types of Cochlear Hypoplasia

Type I (Bud-Like Cochlea)

The cochlea is like a small bud, round or ovoid in shape, arising from the IAC (Fig. 6.6a). Internal architecture is severely deformed; modiolus and interscalar septa cannot be identified.

Type II (Cystic Hypoplastic Cochlea)

The cochlea has smaller dimensions with defective modiolus and interscalar septa, but with normal external outline (Fig. 6.6b). There may be complete absence of modiolus creating a wide connection with the IAC, making gusher and

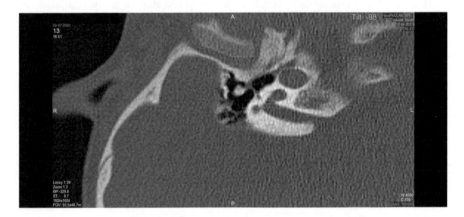

Fig. 6.6a Hypoplasia type I (bud-like cochlea)

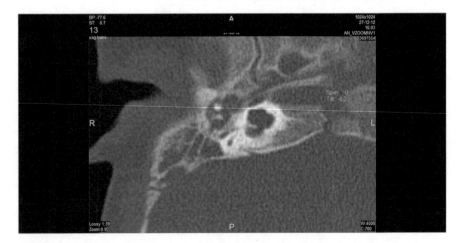

Fig. 6.6b Hypoplasia type II (cystic hypoplastic cochlea)

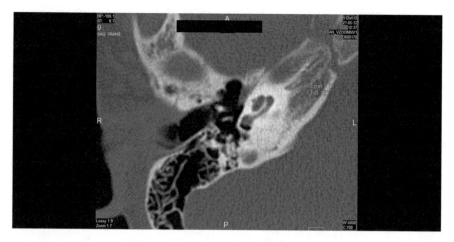

Fig. 6.6c Hypoplasia type III (cochlea with less than two turns)

misplacement of CI electrode into IAC possible. The vestibular aqueduct may be enlarged and the vestibule may be dilated.

Type III (Cochlea with Less Than Two Turns)

The cochlea has fewer turns (i.e., less than two turns) with a short modiolus. The overall length of the interscalar septa is reduced. The internal (modiolus, interscalar septa) and external outlines are similar to that of a normal cochlea, but the dimensions are smaller and number of turns are fewer (Fig. 6.6c). The vestibule and the semicircular canals are usually hypoplastic. The cochlear aperture may be hypoplastic or aplastic.

Type IV (Cochlea with Hypoplastic Middle and Apical Turns)

The cochlea has a normal basal turn, but middle and apical turns are severely hypoplastic and located anterior and medially rather than in their normal central position (Figs. 6.6d and 6.6e). The labyrinthine segment of the facial nerve is usually located anterior to the cochlea rather than in its normal location.

Most probably developmental arrest of membranous labyrinth in CH-III occurs between 6 and 8 weeks, resulting in a cochlea whose dimensions are smaller than normal, with normal internal architecture. In CH-IV arrest in the membranous labyrinth must be between 10 and 20th week, after the basal turn reaches full size, but before the middle and apical turns enlarge to their normal dimensions.

In CH-I and CH-II, there is arrested development of the internal architecture in addition to a small-sized cochlea. In CH-I cochlear duct length must have stopped earlier than normal. Defective modiolar and endosteal development is

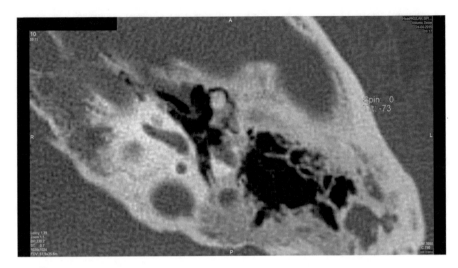

Fig. 6.6d Hypoplasia type IV (cochlea with hypoplastic middle and apical turns)

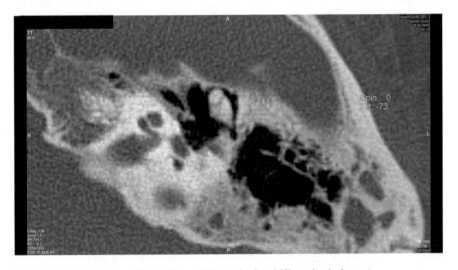

Fig. 6.6e Hypoplasia type IV (cochlea with hypoplastic middle and apical turns)

most probably due to defective vascular supply from the IAC. The main cochlear artery must be defective, resulting in defective endosteal development with an absent modiolus and ISS.

CH-II is better developed than CH-I. The outline of CH-II resembles that of a normal cochlea. It is round or ovoid with a partial modiolar defect. The modiolar base is normal, showing that only the internal radiating arteriole from the main cochlear artery may be defective, while the cochlear ramus of the vestibulocochlear artery supplies the base of the modiolus.

Management

Decision-making in patients with cochlear hypoplasia may be challenging. They may present with a range of different thresholds on audiometric testing. Decision-making about the amplification options may be difficult, particularly in patients with a hypoplastic cochlear nerve. Patients with mild to moderate hearing loss can be habilitated with hearing aids and have near normal to normal language development. The majority of cochlear hypoplasia patients have severe to profound hearing loss where a CI would be a reasonable option, if they have a cochlear nerve. During surgery, facial nerve malposition is to be expected due to associated semicircular abnormalities (particularly lateral semicircular canal). If hypoplastic cochlea is small, the promontory may not have the usual protuberance, and it may be difficult to identify promontory and round window through the facial recess. In these situations, an additional transcanal approach may be necessary to expose the hypoplastic cochlea. The thinner and shorter electrodes should be used in order to obtain full insertion.

Some patients have cochlear aperture aplasia with cochlear nerve aplasia, and thus an ABI would be the best hearing habilitative option. Other patients with cochlear hypoplasia have hypoplastic cochlear nerves. The best option in these cases is to perform CI in the side with better cochlear nerve. If there is limited hearing and language development, an ABI should be considered for the contralateral side.

Some cases of hypoplasia (particularly hypoplasia type IV) may have pure conductive or mixed hearing loss in which the conductive component is due to stapedial fixation. They may benefit from stapedotomy. This can be done in childhood and can result in better oral language development with or without hearing aid usage depending on the bone conduction levels.

6.1.7 Large Vestibular Aqueduct (LVA)

This describes the presence of an enlarged vestibular aqueduct (i.e., the midpoint between posterior labyrinth and operculum is larger than 1.5 mm) in the presence of a normal cochlea, vestibule, and semicircular canals.

Audiological presentation and management is similar to that of IP-II.

6.1.8 Cochlear Aperture Abnormalities

6.1.8.1 Definition and Radiology

The cochlear aperture (CA), cochlear fossette, or cochlear nerve canal transmits the cochlear nerve from the cochlea to IAC. This can be visualized in the mid-modiolar view as well as coronal sections on HRCT (Fig. 6.7a).

The cochlear aperture is considered hypoplastic (Fig. 6.7b) if the width is less than 1.4 mm [22]. The CA is considered to be aplastic when the canal is completely replaced by bone or there is no canal on the mid-modiolar view (Fig. 6.7c).

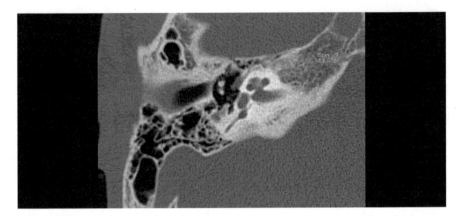

Fig. 6.7a Normal cochlear aperture

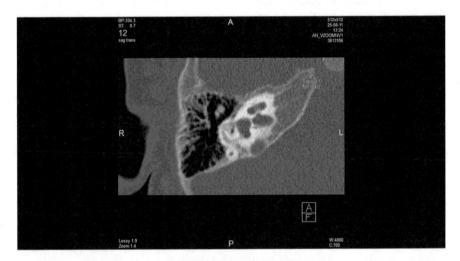

Fig. 6.7b Cochlear aperture stenosis

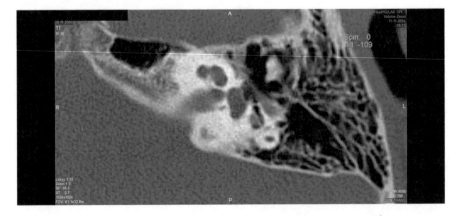

Fig. 6.7c Cochlear aperture aplasia

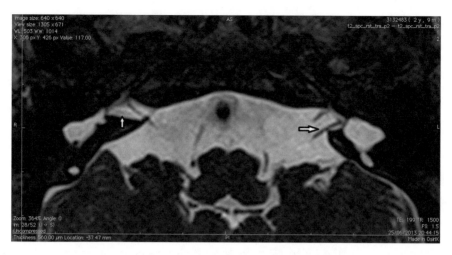

Fig. 6.8d Hypoplastic cochleovestibular nerve (*vertical arrow*) and normal cochleovestibular nerve (*horizontal arrow*)

CA aplasia is typically accompanied by cochlear nerve aplasia. CN may be hypoplastic (Fig. 6.7d) or aplastic when CA is hypoplastic. CA hypoplasia and aplasia can also be observed in a normal cochlea.

CA abnormalities may be accompanied by a narrow IAC on HRCT. The IAC is considered narrow if the width of the midpoint of the IAC is smaller than 2.5 mm (Fig. 6.8d). Narrow IAC can accompany other malformations or with a normal cochlea. In cases of narrow IAC, MRI should be obtained to demonstrate if CN is normal, aplastic, or hypoplastic. Axial and sagittal oblique high T2-weighted images (i.e., CISS, FIESTA, etc.) are necessary for this purpose. On sagittal oblique MR sections, four distinct nerves can be visualized in the IAC (Fig. 6.8e). In CN aplasia, no nerve can be identified in the anterior inferior part of the IAC (Fig. 6.8f).

6.1.8.2   Audiological Findings

Severe to profound SNHL is usually present. As the cochlea is normal, otoacoustic emissions (OAE) may be present, and the child may pass newborn hearing screening if automated ABR is not obtained. Their hearing loss is typically discovered later on in childhood based on the family's concerns of lack of sound awareness and language development. If the newborn screening protocol involves OAE and automated ABR, this malformation can be diagnosed during infancy. Diagnostic audiological evaluation will reveal profound hearing loss.

6.1.8.3 Management

Hearing aids usually do not provide sufficient amplification in patients with CA hypoplasia and aplasia. In patients with bilateral hypoplastic CA with hypoplastic cochlear nerve, hearing aid trial is necessary. If this does not provide adequate functional hearing, these patients usually become candidates for CI. The family should be counseled that if CI does not provide sufficient hearing in terms of auditory perception, contralateral ABI may be necessary to achieve improved audiologic and language outcomes.

In CA aplasia, ABI is indicated as first-line therapy.

6.2 Cochlear Nerve Abnormalities

The classification of cochleovestibular nerve is also important in the management of IEMs.

6.2.1 Normal Cochlear Nerve (CN)

It is important to trace the CN until it enters the cochlea on lower axial sections passing through the IAC (Fig. 6.8a). On parasagittal sections, there is a separate CN located in the anterior inferior part of the IAC, entering the cochlea (Fig. 6.8b). The size of the cochlear nerve is similar in size when compared with the CN on the contralateral normal side. According to Casselman et al. [23] on parasagittal view, the size of the CN is larger than the ipsilateral FN.

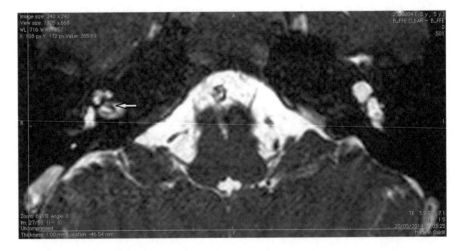

Fig. 6.8a Normal cochlear nerve, axial view

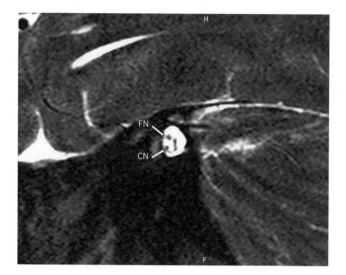

Fig. 6.8b   Normal cochlear nerve, parasagittal view

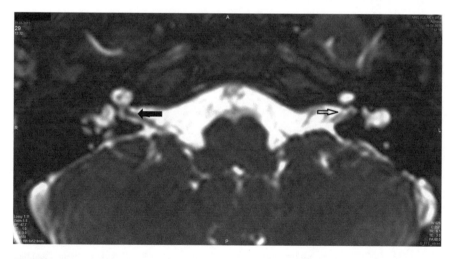

Fig. 6.8c   Normal cochlear nerve on the right (*black arrow*) and hypoplastic cochlear nerve on the left (*white arrow*)

6.2.2   Hypoplastic CN

There is a separate CN, but the size is less than the contralateral normal CN or ipsi-lateral normal facial nerve (Fig. 6.8c).

6.2.3   Absent CN

There is no nerve in the anteroinferior part of the IAC. This is definitely present in cochlear aplasia. It can also be seen in cochlear aperture hypoplasia and aplasia.

6.2.4   Normal CVN

Normally cochlear and vestibular nerves originate at the brainstem together forming the CVN. CVN then separates into CN and superior and inferior vestibular nerves in the IAC. In cases of common cavity, CVN enters the cavity without separating into individual nerves. With radiological precision at the present time, it is impossible to determine the cochlear fiber content in the CVN, but if the size is 1.5–2 times as much as the ipsilateral FN or similar to contralateral normal CVN, it can be accepted as normal (Fig. 6.8d).

6.2.5   Hypoplastic CVN

If CVN is smaller than contralateral CVN or ipsilateral FN, it can be accepted as hypoplastic (Fig. 6.8d). CVN hypoplasia is particularly important in CC.

6.2.6   Absent CVN

In case of Michel deformity with absent IAC, CVN is also absent. Only FN can be identified.

References

1. Sennaroglu L. Cochlear implantation in inner ear malformations – a review article. Cochlear Implants Int. 2010;11(1):4–41.
2. Sennaroglu L, YE, Sennaroglu G, Ozgen B. Management of inner ear malformations. In: Sataloff RT, editor. Sataloff's comprehensive textbook of otolaryngology. JP Medical Publishers; 2015. p. 91–106.
3. Sennaroglu L, Ozkan HB, Aslan F. Impact of cochleovestibular malformations in treating children with hearing loss. Audiol Neuro Otol. 2013;18:23–7.
4. Sennaroglu L. Histopathology of inner ear malformations: do we have enough evidence to explain pathophysiology? Cochlear Implants Int. 2016;17:3–20.
5. Ozgen B, et al. Complete labyrinthine aplasia: clinical and radiologic findings with review of the literature. AJNR Am J Neuroradiol. 2009;30(4):774–80.

6. Donaldson JA, Duckert, Lambert, Rubel EW, editors. Surgical anatomy of the temporal bone. 4th ed. New York: Raven Press; 1992.
7. Sennaroglu L, Sennaroglu G, Atay G. Auditory brainstem implantation in children. Curr Otorhinolaryngol Rep. 2013;1:80–91.
8. McElveen Jr JT, et al. Cochlear implantation in common cavity malformations using a transmastoid labyrinthotomy approach. Laryngoscope. 1997;107(8):1032–6.
9. Sennaroglu L, Saatci I. A new classification for cochleovestibular malformations. Laryngoscope. 2002;112(12):2230–41.
10. Sennaroglu L, Saatci I. Unpartitioned versus incompletely partitioned cochleae: radiologic differentiation. Otol Neurotol. 2004;25(4):520–9; discussion 529.
11. Phelps PD, King A, Michaels L. Cochlear dysplasia and meningitis. Am J Otol. 1994;15(4):551–7.
12. Shetty PG, et al. Cerebrospinal fluid otorhinorrhea in patients with defects through the lamina cribrosa of the internal auditory canal. AJNR Am J Neuroradiol. 1997;18(3):478–81.
13. Syal R, Tyagi I, Goyal A. Cerebrospinal fluid otorhinorrhea due to cochlear dysplasias. Int J Pediatr Otorhinolaryngol. 2005;69(7):983–8.
14. Sennaroglu L. Cochlear implantation in inner ear malformations – a review article. Cochlear Implants Int. 2009.
15. Lo WW. What is a 'Mondini' and what difference does a name make? AJNR Am J Neuroradiol. 1999;20(8):1442–4.
16. Nance WE, et al. X-linked mixed deafness with congenital fixation of the stapedial footplate and perilymphatic gusher. Birth Defects Orig Artic Ser. 1971;07(4):64–9.
17. Phelps PD, et al. X-linked deafness, stapes gushers and a distinctive defect of the inner ear. Neuroradiology. 1991;33(4):326–30.
18. Sennaroglu L, Sarac S, Ergin T. Surgical results of cochlear implantation in malformed cochlea. Otol Neurotol. 2006;27(5):615–23.
19. Talbot JM, Wilson DF. Computed tomographic diagnosis of X-linked congenital mixed deafness, fixation of the stapedial footplate, and perilymphatic gusher. Am J Otol. 1994;15(2):177–82.
20. LS. Special article: incomplete partition type III. In: Naito Y, editor. Pediatric ear diseases diagnostic imaging atlas and case reports. Karger; 2013. p. 106–8.
21. Sennaroglu L editor. Special article: incomplete partition type III in pediatric ear diseases diagnostic imaging atlas and case reports. Karger; 2013. p. 106–8.
22. Wilkins A, et al. Frequent association of cochlear nerve canal stenosis with pediatric sensorineural hearing loss. Arch Otolaryngol Head Neck Surg. 2012;138(4):383–8.
23. Casselman JW, et al. Aplasia and hypoplasia of the vestibulocochlear nerve: diagnosis with MR imaging. Radiology. 1997;202(3):773–81.

Chapter 7
Outcome of Cochlear Implantation in Children with Cochlear Nerve Deficiency and/or Inner Ear Malformations

Lee-Suk Kim and Sung Wook Jeong

Abstract Cochlear implantation is a standard treatment for children with severe-to-profound sensorineural hearing loss. Since the introduction of CI more than 30 years ago, considerable progress has been made, and the eligibility criteria have been expanded repeatedly. However, children with inner ear malformations (IEMs) and/or cochlear nerve deficiency (CND) are still regarded as difficult candidates because the inner ear is the site in which cochlear implant electrodes are positioned and the cochlear nerve is the target of electrical stimulation by the cochlear implant.

This review article, which presents the outcomes of CI performed in children with CND and/or IEMs, shows that they can be favorable candidates for CI. In children with CND, meticulous assessment of the status of the cochlear nerve using high-resolution magnetic resonance imaging and electrical auditory brainstem response can help to identify the optimal candidates for CI and to decide whether to proceed with auditory brainstem implant. If a child with IEM is young and has a competent eighth cranial nerve, a favorable speech perception outcome of CI can be expected.

Keywords Cochlear implant • Child • Inner ear malformation • Cochlear nerve deficiency

7.1 Introduction

Cochlear implantation (CI) is a standard treatment for children with severe-to-profound sensorineural hearing loss (SNHL) who receive limited benefit from a hearing aid. The minimum requirements for CI are a patent cochlear lumen for electrode placement and the presence of cochlear nerve fibers to propagate the

L.-S. Kim, M.D., Ph.D. (✉) • S.W. Jeong, M.D., Ph.D.
Department of Otolaryngology-Head and Neck Surgery, College of Medicine,
Dong-A University, 3-1 Dongdaeshin-dong, Seo-gu, Busan 602-715, South Korea
e-mail: klsolkor@chol.com

© Springer Science+Business Media Singapore 2017   87
K. Kaga (ed.), *Cochlear Implantation in Children with Inner Ear Malformation and Cochlear Nerve Deficiency*, Modern Otology and Neurotology,
DOI 10.1007/978-981-10-1400-0_7

auditory signals to the auditory cortex [1]. Therefore, it is of the utmost importance to examine the structure of the cochlear nerve and inner ear prior to performing CI. On some occasions, however, imaging studies allow the detection of cochlear nerve deficiency (CND) and inner ear malformations (IEMs) during evaluation of candidates for CI. These conditions can be associated with a malformed cochlear lumen, decreased spiral ganglion cell survival, and abnormal tonotopic organization and therefore may impact adversely on speech perception abilities after CI [2, 3]. Furthermore, they increase the risk of surgical complications including cerebrospinal fluid (CSF) gusher, electrode misinsertion into the internal auditory canal (IAC), and facial nerve injury [4–9]. Programming of the speech processor can be difficult because of a narrow electrical dynamic range and facial stimulation [10]. For these reasons, meticulous assessment of the structure of the cochlear nerve and inner ear is required prior to the decision to perform CI. This short article reviews the outcomes of CI performed in children with CND and/or IEMs.

7.2   Cochlear Implantation in Children with CND

7.2.1   Introduction to CND

In the early days of performing CI, the main imaging modality for CI candidates was temporal bone computed tomography (TBCT), which focused on assessing the condition of the inner ear, including labyrinthine ossification or congenital malformation, and the experience with magnetic resonance imaging (MRI) was limited [11, 12]. With the improvement of MRI resolution, four nerves in the IAC, the cochlear nerve, facial nerve, and superior and inferior vestibular nerves, can be clearly identified, and CND has been identified as an important cause of congenital SNHL [13].

Most children with CND have severe-to-profound hearing loss that presents as either SNHL or auditory neuropathy spectrum disorder (ANSD) [14, 15]. CND may be present in up to 18 % of children with SNHL [14] and in 30 % of those with ANSD [15]. A higher incidence of CND has been reported in children with IEMs [1, 3], stenosis of the IAC or cochlear nerve canal (CNC) [16, 17], and ANSD [15, 18]. A study including 59 children with IEMs showed that 19.6 % of them had CND and that the severe forms of IEMs such as common cavity and cochlear aplasia were associated with a much higher incidence of CND [1]. Stenosis of the CNC or IAC is also a strong indicator of CND [16, 17, 19]. A study including 54 ears with CND showed that 36 (66.7 %) had CNC stenosis (<1.5 mm) and 25 (46.3 %) had IAC stenosis (<3.0 mm) [16]. In another study including 42 ears with SNHL, none of the 32 ears with normal CNC had CND but 8 of 10 ears with CNC stenosis (<1.5 mm) had CND [17]. About one-third of children with ANSD have been reported to have CND [15, 18]. A study including 14 children with ANSD showed that five children (35.7 %) had CND [18], and another study reported that 15 of 54 children (28 %)

with ANSD had CND [15]. The incidence of CND is low in hearing-impaired children with normal inner ear morphology [3, 17], but on rare occasions, CND can be present in cases where the structure of the inner ear, CNC, and IAC are normal [20].

CND is challenging for the decision-making process about whether to proceed with CI, because this condition may result in very poor speech perception or even anacusis after CI [14, 20].

7.2.2   Diagnosis of CND

The range of CND includes cochlear nerve hypoplasia and cochlear nerve aplasia. CND is diagnosed using MRI of the IAC [21]. The cochlear nerve is considered to be normal if on the MR image it is the same size or larger than the other nerves in the IAC, including the facial nerve and superior and inferior vestibular nerves. The cochlear nerve is considered to be hypoplastic (small) if it is smaller than the other nerves in the IAC and to be aplastic (absent) if it is not seen on MRI [19]. Heavily T2-weighted gradient echo or turbo-spin echo sequences should be used, and images of the axial and parasagittal planes must be acquired with submillimetric slice thickness to assess accurately the size of the cochlear nerve [22].

7.2.3   Outcome of CI in Children with CND

Children with CND meet the audiometric criteria for CI because most of them have severe-to-profound hearing loss [20]. Although there has been a perception that pathology of the cochlear nerve precludes deaf children from receiving CI, the surgery has been performed for children with CND based on the rationale that children with cochlear nerve hypoplasia can benefit from CI [23] and that some children with cochlear nerve aplasia may have cochlear nerve fibers that are below the resolution of current imaging modalities [14].

However, the outcomes of CI performed for children with CND are unreliable and extremely variable [23–27]. A study that reported the outcome of CI performed in six children with CND showed that five of the children could detect only the presence of sounds and one child could understand some common phrases [24]. All the children achieved very poor speech production at grade 2 speech intelligibility rating (SIR). Many studies of CI outcomes in children with CND have shown that the majority of children with CND obtained very limited benefit after CI, such as improved access to environmental sounds, and that only sporadic cases could acquire open-set speech perception and spoken language [23–27]. In children with CND, therefore, CI should be considered carefully after patients and family members have been fully informed about the uncertain speech and language outcomes.

It is very difficult to predict the outcome of CI prior to surgery in children with CND, but high-resolution MRI and electrical auditory brainstem response (EABR) testing can help. A study including 139 implanted children with CND showed that children with cochlear nerve hypoplasia had a good outcome after CI [23]. In that study, the cochlear nerve aplasia group (one-fifth of the children) showed significantly worse scores on categories of auditory performance (CAP) and SIR after CI than the non-CND group. However, no significant difference was noted between the cochlear nerve hypoplasia group (four-fifths of the children) and the non-CND group. Although MRI is the best imaging tool to visualize the cochlear nerve, it may for various reasons not always differentiate cochlear nerve hypoplasia from aplasia [22]. If images are obtained using a thick section, the resolution can be poor, movement artifacts may obscure the images, or a concomitant narrow IAC or CNC may mask the cochlear nerve. To depict accurately the cochlear nerve, submillimetric thin-section images of the axial and parasagittal planes must be acquired using a 3-tesla MRI scanner rather than a 1.5-tesla MRI scanner [28]. In addition to MRI, EABR using intracochlear electrical stimulation can help predict the outcome of CI in children with CND [15, 29]. The ideal method is transtympanic EABR using promontory or round window stimulation performed before surgery, but studies have failed to show a predictive value of preoperative transtympanic EABR on CI outcomes and the status of the cochlear nerve. One study showed that there were no significant differences in speech perception and production between deaf children with a clear promontory EABR wave and those with no wave [30]. The other study reported that promontory EABR was absent in four children with a narrow IAC who were subsequently found during surgery for auditory brainstem implant (ABI) to have thin vestibulocochlear nerves [31]. However, EABR performed during CI surgery using intracochlear electrical stimulation was reported to have predictive value for the speech perception outcomes after CI in children with CND [15, 29] and children with narrow IAC [32]. The information about the prognosis obtained from EABR performed during or very soon after CI surgery in children with CND can assist in the choice of habilitation method and facilitate decision-making about whether to convert to ABI [32].

An ABI should also be considered for children with CND [14, 22, 31]. A report showed that the children with CND who had a poor performance with a CAP score of 2 or less after CI achieved CAP scores of 2–7 after receiving an ABI for the ipsilateral ear [14]. Another report showed that children with CND who received an ABI outperformed those with CND who received CI [33]. However, the surgical risks related to ABI and the much more difficult programming procedure for the ABI must be considered [22, 33]. Furthermore, ABI is recommended for appropriate candidates aged over 18 months [34]. Therefore, for children with CND, it is better to perform CI as early as possible to minimize the period of auditory deprivation. If a child with CI has an aplastic cochlear nerve on MRI and shows no EABR and no auditory progress, a contralateral ABI should be considered [33].

7.3   Cochlear Implantation in Children with IEMs

7.3.1   Introduction to IEMs

The incidence of IEMs in children with congenital SNHL has been reported to range from 20 to 40 % [35–37]. Most IEMs are considered to be the result of arrested and/or aberrant development during the embryogenesis of the inner ear [35]. Single-gene mutations can also cause IEMs, including the SLC26A4 gene mutation that causes an enlarged vestibular aqueduct [38] and the POU3F4 gene mutation that causes incomplete partition type 3 [39].

When CI surgery was first performed, children with IEMs were regarded as poor candidates for CI because of their abnormal tonotopic organization and the increased risks of surgical complications including CSF gusher, facial nerve injury, or electrode misinsertion into the IAC in patients with a defect of the fundus [2–9]. Currently, however, the presence of IEMs is no longer an obstacle to performing CI and achieving favorable speech perception abilities [1, 40]. There have been numerous reports of CI performed in children with IEMs and promising outcomes have been reported [1, 4, 36, 37, 40, 41]. However, children with some severe forms of IEM, including common cavity or cochlear aplasia, are still difficult candidates for CI, and these types of malformation should be carefully assessed [42–44].

7.3.2   Diagnosis and Classification of IEMs

The best modality to depict IEMs is high-resolution TBCT. Most IEMs can be diagnosed without difficulty using axial and coronal TBCT images that are obtained with submillimetric slice thickness. In cases of an extremely malformed inner ear structure, a three-dimensional volume-rendering technique using MR images can help depict the morphology of the inner ear [37].

The most popular classification system for IEMs originated from the study by Jackler et al. [35], who classified IEMs using inner ear images taken by polytomography. In this classification system, congenital bony cochlear malformations are categorized as one of the following: complete labyrinthine aplasia, cochlear aplasia, cochlear hypoplasia, incomplete partition, or common cavity. Incomplete partition and cochlear hypoplasia are classified further into mild and severe forms. Sennaroglu revised this system using TBCT images [45, 46]. Incomplete partition was further classified into incomplete partition types I, II, and III, and cochlear hypoplasia was classified into types I, II, and III.

Recently, a new classification system for IEMs was introduced by Jeong and Kim [1], who simply classified IEMs into four subtypes based on the morphology of the cochlea and modiolus on TBCT: cochleovestibular malformation (CVM) type A in patients with a normal cochlea and normal modiolus, CVM type B in patients with a malformed cochlea and partial modiolus, CVM type C in patients with a malformed cochlea and no modiolus, and CVM type D in patients with no cochlea and no modiolus. This classification system correlates well with cochlear nerve size and speech perception performance after CI.

7.3.3 Outcome of CI in Children with IEMs

Numerous reports of CI outcomes in children with IEMs have been published [4, 36, 37, 41–44]. However, reports using systematic analysis of the outcomes of large numbers of implanted children with IEMs are lacking, and the majority of the reports are based on limited numbers of patients. According to previously published reports, children with mild IEMs such as incomplete partition type II, malformations of the vestibule or semicircular canals, and enlarged vestibular aqueduct are associated with excellent outcomes after CI that are similar to those of implanted children with normal inner ear morphology [6, 37, 41, 47–49]. However, children with severe IEMs, including common cavity or cochlear aplasia, achieve suboptimal and uncertain speech perception abilities, although they can receive benefits from CI [42–44, 48, 49]. Generally speaking, the outcome of CI in children with IEMs can be considered to be negatively correlated with the severity of the IEM.

Recent studies have shown that the age at CI and the status of the cochlear nerve are the most important determinants of speech perception abilities after CI in children with IEMs [1, 40]. A study including 48 children with IEMs showed that there was no significant relationship between the degree of cochlear abnormality and speech perception/language outcomes and that optimum language outcomes were associated with younger age at CI [40]. In another study including 59 children with IEMs who received CI, the speech perception of the children with IEMs was determined by the age at CI and the size of the cochlear nerve, not by the severity of the IEM [1]. Therefore, children with severe IEMs including common cavity or cochlear aplasia can be favorable candidates for CI if they are young and have a competent vestibulocochlear nerve [1, 43, 44]. In a study including three patients with a common cavity, all three achieved useful open-set speech perception. Two, who had a normal CNC or normal vestibulocochlear nerve and received CI at an early age, showed favorable speech perception, although one child with a narrow CNC who received CI at a later age showed a poor outcome [1]. Children with cochlear aplasia can also be candidates for CI, and the surgery can be performed using the method of inserting an electrode array into the vestibule [43, 44]. Favorable speech perception ability can be achieved if the children with cochlear aplasia are implanted at an early age and have favorable vestibulocochlear nerve integrity [43].

7.4   Conclusion

The cochlear implant is a device to stimulate the spiral ganglion, a cluster of cell bodies of cochlear nerve neurons, using an electrode array inserted into the cochlea. Therefore, there is concern that malformation of the cochlear nerve or cochlea can disturb the surgical procedure of CI and prevent patients from achieving optimal speech and language abilities after CI. This brief review of the outcomes of CI performed in children with CND and/or IEMs shows that they can be favorable candidates for CI. Meticulous assessment of the status of the cochlear nerve using high-resolution MRI and EABR can help to identify the optimal candidates for CI and to decide whether to proceed with ABI in children with CND. If a child with IEM is young and has a competent eighth cranial nerve, a favorable speech perception outcome of CI can be expected.

References

1. Jeong SW, Kim LS. A new classification of cochleovestibular malformations and implications for predicting speech perception ability after cochlear implantation. Audiol Neurotol. 2015;20:90–101.
2. Graham JM, Phelps PD, Michaels L. Congenital malformations of the ear and cochlear implantation in children: review and temporal bone report of common cavity. J Laryngol Otol Suppl. 2000;25:1–14.
3. Giesemann AM, Kontorinis G, Jan Z, Lenarz T, Lanfermann H, Goetz F. The vestibulocochlear nerve: aplasia and hypoplasia in combination with inner ear malformations. Eur Radiol. 2012;22:519–24.
4. Adunka OF, Teagle HF, Zdanski CJ, Buchman CA. Influence of an intraoperative perilymph gusher on cochlear implant performance in children with labyrinthine malformations. Otol Neurotol. 2012;33:1489–96.
5. Hoffman RA, Downey LL, Waltzman SB, Cohen NL. Cochlear implantation in children with cochlear malformations. Am J Otol. 1997;18:184–7.
6. Miyamoto RT, Bichey BG, Wynne MK, Kirk KI. Cochlear implantation with large vestibular aqueduct syndrome. Laryngoscope. 2002;112:1178–82.
7. Molter DW, Pate Jr BR, McElveen Jr JT. Cochlear implantation in the congenitally malformed ear. Otolaryngol Head Neck Surg. 1993;108:174–7.
8. Page EL, Eby TL. Meningitis after cochlear implantation in Mondini malformation. Otolaryngol Head Neck Surg. 1997;116:104–6.
9. Tucci DL, Telian SA, Zimmerman-Phillips S, Zwolan TA, Kileny PR. Cochlear implantation in patients with cochlear malformations. Arch Otolaryngol Head Neck Surg. 1995;121:833–8.
10. Lee Y, Jeong SW, Kim LS. MAP optimization as a predictor of cochlear implant outcomes in children with narrow internal auditory canal. Int J Pediatr Otorhinolaryngol. 2012;76:1591–7.
11. Laszig R, Terwey B, Battmer RD, Hesse G. Magnetic resonance imaging (MRI) and high resolution computertomography (HRCT) in cochlear implant candidates. Scand Audiol Suppl. 1988;30:197–200.
12. Harnsberger HR, Dart DJ, Parkin JL, Smoker WR, Osborn AG. Cochlear implant candidates: assessment with CT and MR imaging. Radiology. 1987;164:53–7.

13. McClay JE, Tandy R, Grundfast K, Choi S, Vezina G, Zalzal G, et al. Major and minor temporal bone abnormalities in children with and without congenital sensorineural hearing loss. Arch Otolaryngol Head Neck Surg. 2002;128:664–71.
14. Colletti L, Wilkinson EP, Colletti V. Auditory brainstem implantation after unsuccessful cochlear implantation of children with clinical diagnosis of cochlear nerve deficiency. Ann Otol Rhinol Laryngol. 2013;122:605–12.
15. Walton J, Gibson WP, Sanli H, Prelog K. Predicting cochlear implant outcomes in children with auditory neuropathy. Otol Neurotol. 2008;29:302–9.
16. Yan F, Li J, Xian J, Wang Z, Mo L. The cochlear nerve canal and internal auditory canal in children with normal cochlea but cochlear nerve deficiency. Acta Radiol. 2013;54:292–8.
17. Miyasaka M, Nosaka S, Morimoto N, Taiji H, Masaki H. CT and MR imaging for pediatric cochlear implantation: emphasis on the relationship between the cochlear nerve canal and the cochlear nerve. Pediatr Radiol. 2010;40:1509–16.
18. Jeong SW, Kim LS. Auditory neuropathy spectrum disorder: predictive value of radiologic studies and electrophysiologic tests on cochlear implant outcomes and its radiologic classification. Acta Otolaryngol. 2013;133:714–21.
19. Glastonbury CM, Davidson HC, Harnsberger HR, Butler J, Kertesz TR, Shelton C. Imaging findings of cochlear nerve deficiency. AJNR Am J Neuroradiol. 2002;23:635–43.
20. Adunka OF, Jewells V, Buchman CA. Value of computed tomography in the evaluation of children with cochlear nerve deficiency. Otol Neurotol. 2007;28:597–604.
21. Casselman JW, Offeciers FE, Govaerts PJ, Kuhweide R, Geldof H, Somers T, et al. Aplasia and hypoplasia of the vestibulocochlear nerve: diagnosis with MR imaging. Radiology. 1997;202:773–81.
22. Freeman SR, Stivaros SM, Ramsden RT, O'Driscoll MP, Nichani JR, Bruce IA, et al. The management of cochlear nerve deficiency. Cochlear Implants Int. 2013;14 Suppl 4:S27–31.
23. Wu CM, Lee LA, Chen CK, Chan KC, Tsou YT, Ng SH. Impact of cochlear nerve deficiency determined using 3-dimensional magnetic resonance imaging on hearing outcome in children with cochlear implants. Otol Neurotol. 2015;36:14–21.
24. Vincenti V, Ormitti F, Ventura E, Guida M, Piccinini A, Pasanisi E. Cochlear implantation in children with cochlear nerve deficiency. Int J Pediatr Otorhinolaryngol. 2014;78:912–7.
25. Buchman CA, Teagle HF, Roush PA, Park LR, Hatch D, Woodard J, et al. Cochlear implantation in children with labyrinthine anomalies and cochlear nerve deficiency: implications for auditory brainstem implantation. Laryngoscope. 2011;121:1979–88.
26. Zhang Z, Li Y, Hu L, Wang Z, Huang Q, Wu H. Cochlear implantation in children with cochlear nerve deficiency: a report of nine cases. Int J Pediatr Otorhinolaryngol. 2012;76:1188–95.
27. Young NM, Kim FM, Ryan ME, Tournis E, Yaras S. Pediatric cochlear implantation of children with eighth nerve deficiency. Int J Pediatr Otorhinolaryngol. 2012;76:1442–8.
28. Giesemann AM, Raab P, Lyutenski S, Dettmer S, Bültmann E, Frömke C, et al. Improved imaging of cochlear nerve hypoplasia using a 3-Tesla variable flip-angle turbo spin-echo sequence and a 7-cm surface coil. Laryngoscope. 2014;124:751–4.
29. Yamazaki H, Leigh J, Briggs R, Naito Y. Usefulness of MRI and EABR testing for predicting CI outcomes immediately after cochlear implantation in cases with cochlear nerve deficiency. Otol Neurotol. 2015;36:977–84.
30. Nikolopoulos TP, Mason SM, Gibbin KP, O'Donoghue GM. The prognostic value of promontory electric auditory brain stem response in pediatric cochlear implantation. Ear Hear. 2000;21:236–41.
31. Song MH, Kim SC, Kim J, Chang JW, Lee WS, Choi JY. The cochleovestibular nerve identified during auditory brainstem implantation in patients with narrow internal auditory canals: can preoperative evaluation predict cochleovestibular nerve deficiency? Laryngoscope. 2011;121:1773–9.
32. Song MH, Bae MR, Kim HN, Lee WS, Yang WS, Choi JY. Value of intracochlear electrically evoked auditory brainstem response after cochlear implantation in patients with narrow internal auditory canal. Laryngoscope. 2010;120:1625–31.

33. Colletti L, Colletti G, Mandalà M, Colletti V. The therapeutic dilemma of cochlear nerve deficiency: cochlear or brainstem implantation? Otolaryngol Head Neck Surg. 2014;151:308–14.
34. Sennaroglu L, Colletti V, Manrique M, Laszig R, Offeciers E, Saeed S, et al. Auditory brainstem implantation in children and non-neurofibromatosis type 2 patients: a consensus statement. Otol Neurotol. 2011;32:187–91.
35. Jackler RK, Luxford WM, House WF. Congenital malformations of the inner ear: a classification based on embryogenesis. Laryngoscope. 1987;97 suppl 40:2–14.
36. Papsin BC. Cochlear implantation in children with anomalous cochleovestibular anatomy. Laryngoscope. 2005;115 suppl 106:1–26.
37. Kim LS, Jeong SW, Huh MJ, Park YD. Cochlear implantation in children with inner ear malformations. Ann Otol Rhinol Laryngol. 2006;115:205–14.
38. Reardon W, OMahoney CF, Trembath R, Jan H, Phelps PD. Enlarged vestibular aqueduct: a radiological marker of pendred syndrome, and mutation of the PDS gene. QJM. 2000;93:99–104.
39. Choi BY, An YH, Park JH, Jang JH, Chung HC, Kim AR, et al. Audiological and surgical evidence for the presence of a third window effect for the conductive hearing loss in DFNX2 deafness irrespective of types of mutations. Eur Arch Otorhinolaryngol. 2013;270:3057–62.
40. Dettman S, Sadeghi-Barzalighi A, Ambett R, Dowell R, Trotter M, Briggs R. Cochlear implants in forty-eight children with cochlear and/or vestibular abnormality. Audiol Neurotol. 2011;16:222–32.
41. Eisenman DJ, Ashbaugh C, Zwolan TA, Arts HA, Telian SA. Implantation of the malformed cochlea. Otol Neurotol. 2001;22:834–41.
42. Xia J, Wang W, Zhang D. Cochlear implantation in 21 patients with common cavity malformation. Acta Otolaryngol. 2015;135:459–65.
43. Jeong SW, Kim LS. Cochlear implantation in children with cochlear aplasia. Acta Otolaryngol. 2012;132:910–5.
44. Kontorinis G, Goetz F, Giourgas A, Lanfermann H, Lenarz T, Giesemann AM. Aplasia of the cochlea: radiologic assessment and options for hearing rehabilitation. Otol Neurotol. 2013;34:1253–60.
45. Sennaroglu L, Saatci I. A new classification for cochleovestibular malformations. Laryngoscope. 2002;112:2230–41.
46. Sennaroglu L. Cochlear implantation in inner ear malformations – a review article. Cochlear Implants Int. 2010;11:4–41.
47. Bent 3rd JP, Chute P, Parisier SC. Cochlear implantation in children with enlarged vestibular aqueducts. Laryngoscope. 1999;109(7 Pt 1):1019–22.
48. Woolley AL, Jenison V, Stroer BS, Lusk RP, Bahadori RS, Wippold FJ. Cochlear implantation in children with inner ear malformations. Ann Otol Rhinol Laryngol. 1998;107:492–500.
49. Weber BP, Dillo W, Dietrich B, Maneke I, Bertram B, Lenarz T. Pediatric cochlear implantation in cochlear malformations. Am J Otol. 1998;19:747–53.

Chapter 8
EABR of Inner Ear Malformation and Cochlear Nerve Deficiency After Cochlear Implantation in Children

Shujiro Minami and Kimitaka Kaga

Abstract When cochlear implantation has been performed in a case involving inner ear malformations, it is particularly important to perform objective physiological measurements of the cochlear implant. The inner ear malformations can be divided into categories according to the observation of modiolus deficiency and/or cochlear nerve deficiency (CND). CND severity can be categorized in one of three ways, according to the MRI findings: (1) a hypoplastic cochlear nerve, (2) the absence of cochlear nerve, and (3) the absence of vestibulocochlear nerve. EABR is a reliable and effective way of objectively confirming device function and implant responsiveness of the peripheral auditory neurons up to the level of the brainstem in cases of inner ear malformation. EABR can often be recorded in cases in which the presence of excessive stimulus artifacts precludes the successful acquisition of ECAP, such as in cases with modiolus deficiency cochlea. This chapter presents cases with or without modiolus deficiency, depending on the severity of cochlear nerve deficiency, and describes their EABR characteristics. Vestibular simulated EABR is also shown, demonstrating the interactions between vestibular and auditory pathways.

Keywords EABR • Modiolus deficiency • Cochlear nerve deficiency

S. Minami (✉)
Division of Otolaryngology, National Tokyo Medical Center,
2-5-1 higashigaoka, Meguro-ku, Tokyo 152-8902, Japan
e-mail: shujirominami@me.com

K. Kaga
National Institute of Sensory Organs, National Tokyo Medical Center,
2-5-1 Higashigaoka, Meguro-Ku, Tokyo 152-8902, Japan

Center for Speech and Hearing Disorders, International University of Health
and Welfare Clinic, 2600-6 Kitakanemaru, Ohtawara, Tochigi 324-0011, Japan

© Springer Science+Business Media Singapore 2017　　　　　　　　　97
K. Kaga (ed.), *Cochlear Implantation in Children with Inner Ear Malformation
and Cochlear Nerve Deficiency*, Modern Otology and Neurotology,
DOI 10.1007/978-981-10-1400-0_8

8.1   Introduction

When inner ear malformations are present, it is particularly important to perform objective measurements of the cochlear implant (CI), as these measurements will show whether the electrodes are appropriately positioned and whether there is initial failure of the device during surgery. These measurements are also useful for predicting the audiological outcomes after CI implantation, for assisting the speech processor fitting when behavioral results are difficult to obtain, and for characterizing the pathophysiology of hearing loss. The different ways of objectively measuring CI function can be divided into those that measure nonphysiological variables and those that measure physiological variables. Objective nonphysiological assessment tools include those that measure electrode-specific voltage, impedance, and electrical field patterns across the array. These provide insights into the properties of the surrounding tissue, the electrode–tissue interface, and the path of current flow and help to identify electrode failures [1]. However, these tools are not used to assess the physiological function of the auditory pathway. Physiological objective assessment tools measure various aspects of the auditory responses to electrical stimulation through a CI. These include electrically evoked stapedial reflexes [2], electrically evoked compound action potentials (ECAPs) [3], electrically evoked auditory brainstem responses (EABRs) [4], electrically evoked auditory middle latency responses [5], and electrically evoked auditory cortical potentials [6]. ECAP can be recorded quickly and easily without the need for surface or scalp electrodes and is probably the most widely used measure in clinical settings. In contrast, while EABR recordings require the placement of surface electrodes, they can provide information about the auditory pathway up to the level of the brainstem [7].

The inner ear malformations can be categorized according to the type of modiolus deficiency and/or cochlear nerve deficiency (CND), if any. The modiolus present type includes enlarged vestibular aqueduct (EVA), incomplete partition type II (IP-II), and cochlear hypoplasia type III (CH-III). The modiolus absent type includes common cavities (CC) and incomplete partition type I (IP-I). CND can be divided into three categories, according to the MRI findings (Fig. 8.1a–d): (1) a hypoplastic cochlear nerve; cochlear nerve can be identified, but is smaller than facial nerve; (2) the absence of cochlear nerve; vestibulocochlear nerve can be identified but cochlear nerve cannot be separated; and (3) the absence of vestibulocochlear nerve; vestibulocochlear nerve cannot be confirmed at all. The present chapter shows cases of each type, describing their EABR characteristics.

Fig. 8.1 Reformatted parasagittal oblique MRI images. (**a**) A normal cochlear nerve of larger diameter than the facial nerve. *F* facial nerve, *C* cochlear nerve, *SV* super. (**b**) A hypoplastic cochlear nerve of smaller diameter than the facial nerve (*red triangle*). (**c**) Facial and vestibulocochlear (*red triangle*) nerves are identified, but cochlear nerve is not separated. (**d**) Absence of vestibulocochlear nerve. Only facial nerve is recognized

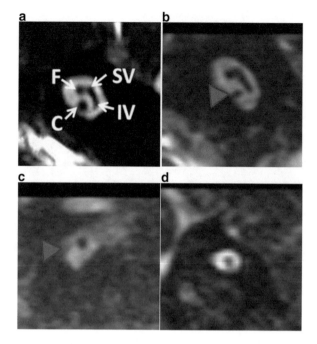

8.2 Measurement and Reading of EABR

8.2.1 Measurement of Intracochlear EABR

EABRs were recorded on electrodes within the cochlea. The responses were recorded with the Neuropack (Nihon Kohden Co., Tokyo, Japan) electrodiagnostic system and were triggered externally by the stimulus output of each CI company's software and the interface unit. The interface unit was also connected to a stock speech processor and the subject's headpiece; the stimulus signal was transmitted across the skin to the implanted device. The electrically evoked brainstem potentials were recorded by using needle electrodes placed on the forehead (different electrode), the nape of the neck (indifferent electrode), and the contralateral earlobe (reference electrode). The recording of electrical activity included two or three replications of 1000 sweeps at each stimulus level with a time window of 10 ms for each stimulus condition. Frequency cutoffs of 100 and 1000 Hz were used. The pulse duration was set to 30 ms and the stimulation amplitude for a single recording fell from high to low current. If no response was detected, pulse duration was increased.

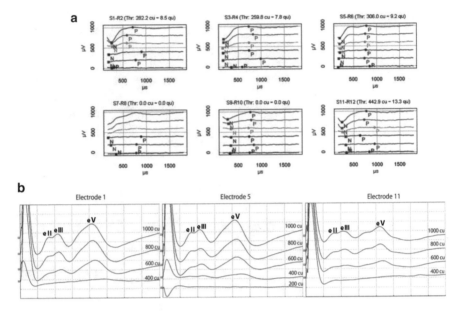

Fig. 8.2 (**a**) ECAP waves of case no. 1. (**b**) EABR waves of case no. 1

8.2.2 *EABR Waves of Patients Without Inner Ear Malformation*

8.2.2.1 Case No. 1

In this case, hearing loss was found by newborn hearing screening. Congenital cytomegalovirus infection was confirmed by polymerase chain reaction for cytomegalovirus DNA in his umbilical cord. CT and MRI studies showed normal inner ear structure. He was fitted with hearing aids bilaterally, but his hearing loss progressed to profound sensorineural hearing loss. At the age of 3 years, he underwent implantation with a CONCERTO Flex28 (MED-EL, Innsbruck, Austria). All electrodes were inserted, and further assessment via telemetry showed good ECAP and EABR responses via the cochlear implant (Fig. 8.2a, b). After cochlear implantation, his hearing recovered well, and he achieved an IT-MAIS score of 34 at 6 months after implantation.

8.2.2.2 Comment

The basal electrodes have higher thresholds and longer wave eV latencies than the apical and middle electrodes. It may be that the higher thresholds and longer wave eV latencies of the most basal electrodes are the result of the greater distance from the neural elements compared to the more apical electrodes, which are located further along the scala tympani. According to our series, the mean wave eIII latencies of the ears without a malformation for apical and basal electrodes were 2.29 ± 0.22 and 2.40 ± 0.24 ms, and the mean wave eV latencies of the ears without a malformation for apical and basal electrodes were 4.26 ± 0.40 and 4.55 ± 0.32 ms [8]. All children without malformations had EABR wave eV latencies of less than 5 ms. The patients were divided into three groups according to their EABR responses. The *typical* response group included all patients showing reproducible wave eV responses with EABR eV latencies of less than 5 ms. The *atypical* response group was defined as those patients who presented with reproducible wave eV responses that were measured in only a limited number of electrodes and/or that showed EABR eV latencies of more than 5 ms pulse duration. In the *no* response group, no identifiable wave eV responses could be seen in any of the electrodes, even with longer pulse duration.

8.3 EABR Waves of Patients with Modiolus Present Type of Inner Ear Malformation

8.3.1 Modiolus Present and Cochlear Nerve Present Type

8.3.1.1 Case No. 2

This is a case of congenital progressive hearing loss with bilateral enlarged vestibular aqueduct (EVA) (Fig. 8.3a, b). SLC26A4 mutations were confirmed. At the age of 3 years, she underwent implantation with a CONCERTO Flex soft (MED-EL) in her right ear. All electrodes were inserted, and further assessment via telemetry showed good ECAP and EABR responses via the cochlear implant (Fig. 8.3c). After cochlear implantation, her hearing recovered well.

8.3.1.2 Comment

The presence of enlarged vestibular aqueduct (EVA) in the presence of normal cochlea, vestibule, and SCCs is a typical case of modiolus present and cochlear nerve present type of inner ear malformation. This type of inner ear malformation shows as good EABR and CI performance as those without malformation. In the cochlear malformation cases in which the modiolus was present, the basal electrodes have higher thresholds and longer wave eV latencies than the apical and middle electrodes. These are similar threshold and latency patterns to those observed in the patients without malformations.

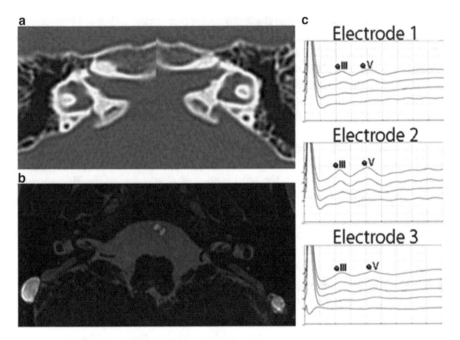

Fig. 8.3 (a) Axial computed tomography imaging study showing enlarged vestibular aqueduct malformation. (b) Axial MRI study showing enlarged vestibular aqueduct malformation and normal cochlear nerves. (c) EABR waves of case no. 2

8.3.2 Modiolus Present and Cochlear Nerve Deficiency Type

8.3.2.1 Case No. 3

This child was 10 years old and had progressive hearing loss (Fig. 8.4a). She has a very thin cochlear nerve canal in CT (Fig. 8.4b), and her cochlear nerves could not be seen on MRI (Fig. 8.4c), but she had obvious auditory response on both ears. She had cochlear implantation (MED-EL CONCERTO Flex soft) on the left ear. Her ECAP showed a threshold at 600 CU (current unit) with a 30-ms pulse duration (Fig. 8.4d), which is the usual pulse width. Meanwhile, her EABR threshold was 800 CU with a 55 ms pulse duration (Fig. 8.4e), which means that we need to nearly double the intensity to obtain the EABR threshold as compared with ECAP. Now, her category of auditory performance (CAP) score is 6, and she is very satisfied with CI.

8.3.2.2 Comment

Even the patient has cochlear nerve deficiency, if she has obvious auditory response with hearing aids, she can be a good indication for cochlear implantation. Because obvious auditory response implies that the cochlear nerve is functionable. Cochlear nerve canal stenosis cases have normal spiral ganglion cells, so ECAP shows good

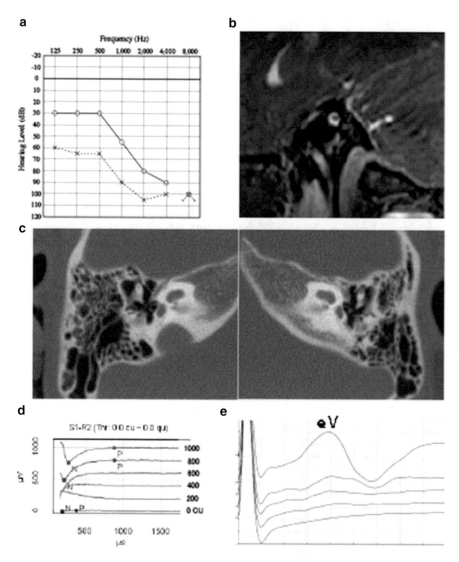

Fig. 8.4 (**a**) Pure tone audiometric result for case no. 3 before cochlear implantation. (**b**) Parasagittal oblique MRI study showing the absence of cochlear nerve. (**c**) Axial computed tomography imaging study showing cochlear nerve canal stenosis. (**d**) ECAP waves of case no. 3. (**e**). EABR waves of case no. 3

responses with the usual intensity. However, because a high intensity is needed to go through the thin auditory nerve, the EABR threshold is high. It may be better to use modiolar-hugging electrodes, because peri-modiolar electrode placement reduces the spread of excitation of CI stimulation. These reduced nerve stimulation thresholds may result in improved speech discrimination by implant users with modiolus presence and cochlear nerve deficiency.

8.4   EABR Waves of Patients with Modiolus Absent Type of Inner Ear Malformation

8.4.1   Modiolus Absent and Vestibulocochlear Nerve Present Type

8.4.1.1   Case No. 4

This child has congenital profound hearing loss with bilateral common cavity (CC) malformation (Fig. 8.5a). He underwent cochlear implantation with PULSAR Standard (MED-EL) at 2 years old in his right ear and CONCERTO Standard (MED-EL) at 4 years 8 months old in his left ear. In the right ear, no ECAP response and variable EABR responses were obtained; in the left ear, variable ECAP and EABR responses were obtained (Fig. 8.5b, c). His IT-MAIS score was 35 at 1 year after first implantation.

8.4.1.2   Comment

The type of cochlear malformation characterized by modiolus absence and vestibulo-cochlear nerve presence is CC or incomplete partition type I (IP-I) with open fundus of the internal auditory canal (IAC). ECAP recordings depend largely on spinal

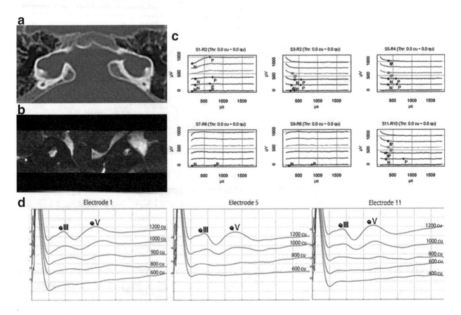

Fig. 8.5 (**a**) Axial computed tomography imaging study showing common cavity malformation. (**b**) Parasagittal oblique MRI study showing vestibulocochlear and facial nerves. (**c**) ECAP waves of case no. 4. (**d**) EABR waves of case no. 4

ganglion cells, which are very often defective in modiolus deficiency-type malformed cochlea. EABR can be obtained in modiolus deficiency-type implant users because the measures are not dependent on the implant having telemetry capabilities and because the wave eV of EABR, which occurs at a later latency than ECAP, is easier to isolate from the stimulus artifacts. The cochlear malformation cases with modiolus deficiency did not exhibit threshold and latency differences between electrodes. The auditory nerve tissues in modiolus deficiency malformations are supposed to be in the inner ear wall, and so the distances from each electrode to the auditory nerve tissue should not be different in modiolus deficiency-type malformations.

8.4.2 Modiolus Absent and Vestibulocochlear Nerve Deficiency

8.4.2.1 Case No. 5

This patient was 1 year and 6 months old and has common cavity with very narrow internal auditory canal on both sides (Fig. 8.6a). Only the facial nerves were recognized by the MRI (Fig. 8.6b). The auditory response with hearing aids was vague, but the damped-rotational chair test (DRCT) showed normal vestibular function (Fig. 8.6c). She had cochlear implantation in the left ear. The intracochlear EABR during surgery showed typical good responses at all electrodes (Fig. 8.6d). Now, she shows obvious auditory response with CI and takes auditory verbal education.

8.4.2.2 Comment

This type of malformation is challenging. Some doctors may say this is a case of cochlear aplasia with enlarged vestibule. We think good vestibular functions in the cases of comorbidity of common cavity and narrow internal auditory canal can be an indication for CI. In the case of internal auditory canal stenosis, vestibular evaluation helps us to determine the neural connection between the inner ear and the brain. It is possible that vestibular nerves can obtain the function of auditory nerve via auditory stimulation plasticity. Amphibians and reptiles are able to hear without cochlea. Smith reported interactions between the vestibular nucleus and the dorsal cochlear nucleus [9]. The next case (no. 6) demonstrated the possibility of these interactions.

8.5 Vestibular Simulated EABR

8.5.1 Case No. 6

This patient suffered bilateral profound hearing loss at age 3 as a result of meningitis. He underwent cochlear implantation with Concerto Flex28 (MED-EL) at 20 years old in his left ear. He had stage I cochlear ossification; all electrodes were

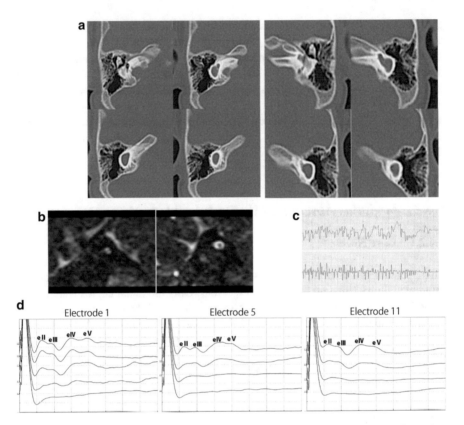

Fig. 8.6 (**a**) Axial computed tomography imaging study showing common cavity malformation and severe internal auditory canal stenosis. (**b**) Parasagittal oblique MRI study showing only facial nerves. (**c**) DRCT response of case no. 5. (**d**) EABR waves of case no. 5

wrongly inserted to vestibule and semicircular canals (Fig. 8.7a). After we found the wrong insertion, he underwent reoperation, and his hearing recovered well. Figure 8.7b showed vestibular simulated EABR in wrong insertion.

8.5.2 Comment

This is an unexpected case. The EABR in the vestibule and semicircular insertion showed reproducible wave eIII, eIV, and eV responses with similar latencies to case no. 5. Previous studies showed direct projections from the vestibular nerve to the dorsal cochlear nucleus (DCN) [9, 10]. These results suggest that the lateral vestibular nucleus (LVN) projects directly to the DCN, some of which may also receive direct projections from the vestibular nerve. Thus, vestibular and auditory information processing may be intimately connected.

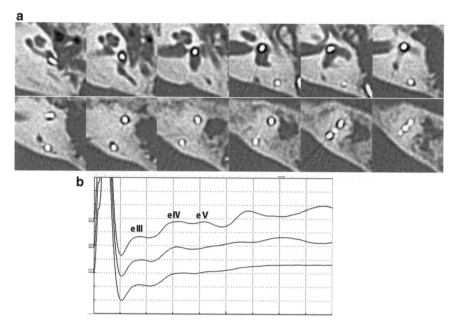

Fig. 8.7 (**a**) Axial computed tomography imaging study showing wrong insertion to vestibule and semicircular canals. (**b**) EABR waves of case no. 6 in wrong insertion

8.6   Our Series of Cochlear Nerve Deficiency

Table 8.1 shows our 20 cases of CND who had CI surgery. We evaluated our 20 cases of CNDs by CT and MRI, vestibular functions (damped-rotational chair test), and intracochlear EABR during CI surgery. 65 % of CNDs had comorbidity of cochlear malformation, 25 % incomplete partition (IP)-I, 20 % cochlear hypoplasia, 15 % common cavity, and 5 % IP-II. On MRI one case showed a thin cochlear nerve, and 60 % showed the absence of cochlear nerves but the presence of vestibulocochlear nerves. The absence of vestibulocochlear nerves is found in 25 % of CNDs. With vestibular function tests before CI surgery, 60 % of CNDs showed normal, 25 % poor, and 10 % no response. In the cases with vestibulocochlear nerves found on MRI, 67 % showed typical EABR, while in the cases with no vestibulocochlear nerve, just one showed typical EABR. 64 % of good vestibular function cases showed typical EABR, while only 29 % of poor or no vestibular function cases showed typical EABR. In the cases with thin or absent cochlear nerves, the vestibulocochlear nerves found on MRI and obvious auditory responses with hearing aids are possible indications for CI. Even if the imaging studies show an absence of vestibulocochlear nerves, the cases with good vestibular functions can be indicated for CI, because vestibular evaluation helps us to determine the neural connection between the inner ear and the brain. Not only imaging evaluations but also evaluations by auditory response and vestibular function are important for CI

Table 8.1 Our 20 cases of cochlear nerve deficiency

Pt	CI age (years)	Cochlear malformation	Modiolus	MRI	DRCT pre-CI	EABR
1	4	No	Present	Absence of cochlear nerve	Normal	Atypical
2	2	IP-I	Absent	Absence of cochlear nerve	Normal	Typical
3	5	Cochlear hypoplasia	Present	Absence of cochlear nerve	N/A	Typical
4	2	IP-I	Absent	Absence of cochlear nerve	No response	Typical
5	2	No	Present	Absence of cochlear nerve	Normal	Typical
6	2	Common cavity	Absent	Absence of cochlear nerve	Poor	Typical
7	3	IP-I	Absent	Absence of cochlear nerve	Poor	Atypical
8	2	Cochlear hypoplasia	Present	Absence of cochlear nerve	Normal	Typical
9	2	Cochlear hypoplasia	Present	Absence of cochlear nerve	No response	Atypical
10	10	No	Present	Absence of cochlear nerve	Normal	Typical
11	6	IP-II	Present	Hypoplastic cochlear nerve	Normal	Typical
12	2	IP-I	Absent	Absence of cochlear nerve	Normal	N/A
13	4	Common cavity	Absent	Absence of cochlear nerve	Normal	Typical
14	2	No	Present	Absence of cochlear nerve	Normal	Atypical
15	4	No	Present	Absence of vestibulocochlear nerve	Poor	No response
16	1	Common cavity	Absent	Absence of vestibulocochlear nerve	Normal	Typical
17	11	No	Present	Absence of vestibulocochlear nerve	Normal	No response
18	1	IP-I	Absent	Absence of cochlear nerve	Poor	Atypical
19	2	No	Present	Absence of vestibulocochlear nerve	Normal	Atypical
20	26	Cochlear hypoplasia	Present	Absence of vestibulocochlear nerve	Poor	Atypical

indication of CNDs. Even in typical EABR cases, some cases show poor auditory performance with CI because of developmental disability. It is difficult to evaluate developmental disability in early childhood, and so we should pay considerable attention to this comorbidity with developmental disability.

References

1. Carlson ML, Archibald DJ, Dabade TS, Gifford RH, Neff BA, Beatty CW, et al. Prevalence and timing of individual cochlear implant electrode failures. Otol Neurotol. 2010;31(6):893–8. doi:10.1097/MAO.0b013e3181d2d697.
2. Lorens A, Walkowiak A, Piotrowska A, Skarzynski H, Anderson I. ESRT and MCL correlations in experienced paediatric cochlear implant users. Cochlear Implants Int. 2004;5(1):28–37. doi:10.1002/cii.121.
3. Botros A, Psarros C. Neural response telemetry reconsidered: I. The relevance of ECAP threshold profiles and scaled profiles to cochlear implant fitting. Ear Hear. 2010;31(3):367–79. doi:10.1097/AUD.0b013e3181c9fd86.
4. Bierer JA, Faulkner KF, Tremblay KL. Identifying cochlear implant channels with poor electrode-neuron interfaces: electrically evoked auditory brain stem responses measured with the partial tripolar configuration. Ear Hear. 2011;32(4):436–44. doi:10.1097/AUD.0b013e3181ff33ab.
5. Miller AL, Arenberg JG, Middlebrooks JC, Pfingst BE. Cochlear implant thresholds: comparison of middle latency responses with psychophysical and cortical-spike-activity thresholds. Hear Res. 2001;152(1–2):55–66.
6. Beynon AJ, Snik AF, van den Broek P. Evaluation of cochlear implant benefit with auditory cortical evoked potentials. Int J Audiol. 2002;41(7):429–35.
7. Firszt JB, Chambers RD. Kraus, Reeder RM. Neurophysiology of cochlear implant users I: effects of stimulus current level and electrode site on the electrical ABR, MLR, and N1-P2 response. Ear Hear. 2002;23(6):502–15. doi:10.1097/01.AUD.0000042153.40602.54.
8. Minami SB, Takegoshi H, Shinjo Y, Enomoto C, Kaga K. Usefulness of measuring electrically evoked auditory brainstem responses in children with inner ear malformations during cochlear implantation. Acta Otolaryngol. 2015;135(10):1007–15. doi:10.3109/00016489.2015.1048377.
9. Smith PF. Interactions between the vestibular nucleus and the dorsal cochlear nucleus: implications for tinnitus. Hear Res. 2012;292(1–2):80–2. doi:10.1016/j.heares.2012.08.006.
10. Barker M, Solinski HJ, Hashimoto H, Tagoe T, Pilati N, Hamann M. Acoustic overexposure increases the expression of VGLUT-2 mediated projections from the lateral vestibular nucleus to the dorsal cochlear nucleus. PLoS One. 2012;7(5), e35955. doi:10.1371/journal.pone.0035955.

Chapter 9
Vestibular Neuropathy

Shinichi Iwasaki

Abstract Auditory neuropathy is a disorder which is defined as hearing loss combined with severe abnormalities of auditory brainstem responses (ABRs) in the presence of preserved cochlear outer hair cell function indicated by normal evoked otoacoustic emissions (OAEs) and/or cochlear microphonics. On the other hand, neuropathies of the vestibular nerves have not been commonly recognized. One reason for this situation may be due to ambiguity in the definition of vestibular neuropathy, since until recently there were no vestibular tests such as ABR or DPOAE which can discriminate between labyrinthine and retrolabyrinthine lesions. Another reason is that some patients with bilateral vestibular dysfunction do not express symptoms of a vestibular disorder. Currently, vestibular neuropathy is usually diagnosed from circumstantial evidence. This chapter describes (1) vestibular dysfunction in patients with auditory neuropathy, (2) vestibular involvement in other neuropathies, and (3) retrolabyrinthine involvement in idiopathic bilateral vestibulopathy, in the literature as well as in our experience. This review concludes that many patients with auditory neuropathy or other neuropathies also have bilateral vestibular dysfunction.

Keywords Auditory neuropathy • Vestibular • Caloric • Vestibular evoked myogenic potentials

9.1 Introduction

Auditory neuropathy is a disorder which is defined as hearing loss in the presence of preserved cochlear outer hair cell function indicated by normal evoked otoacoustic emissions (OAEs) and/or cochlear microphonics combined with severe abnormalities of auditory brainstem responses (ABRs), suggesting hearing loss caused by

S. Iwasaki, M.D. (✉)
Department of Otorhinolaryngology, Head and Neck Surgery, Graduate School of Medicine,
The University of Tokyo, 7-3-1 Hongo, Bunkyo-ku, Tokyo 113-8655, Japan
e-mail: iwashin-tky@umin.ac.jp

© Springer Science+Business Media Singapore 2017
K. Kaga (ed.), *Cochlear Implantation in Children with Inner Ear Malformation and Cochlear Nerve Deficiency*, Modern Otology and Neurotology,
DOI 10.1007/978-981-10-1400-0_9

retrocochlear lesions. After the first descriptions of auditory neuropathy by Starr et al. [1] and Kaga et al. [2], there have been many reports on this disease (for review, see [3]).

On the other hand, neuropathies of the vestibular nerves have not been commonly recognized. One reason for this situation may be ambiguity in the definition of vestibular neuropathy, since until recently there were no vestibular tests such as ABR or DPOAE (distortion product otoacoustic emissions), which were able to discriminate between labyrinthine and retrolabyrinthine lesions. Another reason is that some patients with bilateral vestibular dysfunction do not express symptoms of a vestibular disorder; hence, such patients do not undergo vestibular function tests.

At present, vestibular neuropathy is diagnosed from circumstantial evidence. For example, patients with vestibular dysfunction as well as other neuropathies are usually considered to have vestibular neuropathy. In this chapter, the current status of vestibular neuropathy in the literature is reviewed.

9.2 Auditory Neuropathy with Vestibular Involvement

A proportion of patients with auditory neuropathy have bilateral vestibular dysfunction. Starr et al. [1] described ten patients with auditory neuropathy, three of whom showed horizontal nystagmus on lateral gaze and two others who had absent caloric responses [1]. Additionally, all of these five patients had generalized peripheral neuropathy. The authors suggested the abnormal results of auditory as well as vestibular function tests formed part of a generalized neuropathic disorder affecting both components of the eighth cranial verve.

Kaga et al. [2] also reported on two patients with auditory neuropathy (auditory nerve disease) in the same year [2]. These patients complained of vestibular symptoms, and ice water caloric tests revealed no responses bilaterally in either patient. They attributed the results to a slight involvement of the vestibular organs and brainstem and a possible lesion in the cochlear nerve.

Patients with auditory neuropathy who do not have vestibular symptoms such as imbalance or oscillopsia may nevertheless have vestibular disorders. Fujikawa and Starr [4] performed caloric tests in 14 patients with auditory neuropathy who had not experienced any symptoms of vestibular disorders [4]. Abnormal caloric responses were found in 9 of the 14 patients (64 %), 7 of whom also had peripheral neuropathies. The mean age of the nine patients with vestibular dysfunction (35.6 years) was older than that in patients without vestibular dysfunction (17.8 years). The reason for the lack of vestibular symptoms might have been the bilateral involvement of the dysfunction and a slow rate of vestibular nerve degeneration. Masuda and Kaga [5] reported the chronological deterioration of vestibular function in three patients with auditory neuropathy [5].

Cervical vestibular evoked myogenic potentials (cVEMPs) have been recorded in patients with auditory neuropathy to evaluate the function of the saccule and inferior vestibular nerves [6, 7]. Sheykholeslami et al. [7] reported a bilateral absence of cVEMP responses in three patients with auditory neuropathy but without peripheral neuropathy [7]. Sazgar et al. [6] also recorded cVEMPs in eight patients with auditory neuropathy and showed abnormal cVEMP responses in 13 of 16 ears (81 %): unrepeatable waves in four ears and absent responses in nine ears [6]. These results suggest that auditory neuropathy can involve the inferior vestibular nerve as well as the cochlear nerve.

Histopathological changes in the vestibular nerves in auditory neuropathy have been reported by Starr et al. [8]. They examined the histopathology of the temporal bones in a patient with auditory neuropathy accompanied by mutations in the myelin protein zero (*MPZ*) gene, who had an absence of caloric responses in both ears. They reported a reduction of the number of nerve fibers between the vestibular receptors and the vestibular ganglion despite the normal appearance of the sensory epithelium of the vestibular organs. The number of vestibular ganglion cells was not reduced. Approximately one-third of the laterally projecting vestibular nerve had an irregular beaded appearance, indicating incomplete remyelination of the nerve. Similar changes were also observed in the cochlear nerve and sural nerve in their study. These results suggest that vestibular lesions in auditory neuropathy are mainly caused by axonal disease as part of a generalized neuropathy.

Auditory neuropathy may accompany peripheral neuropathy in a variety of autosomal dominant syndromes as described below. However, mutations in the otoferlin (*OTOF*) gene, the cause of DFNB9 recessive deafness, are implicated in recessive non-syndromic deafness in auditory neuropathy [9]. Otoferlin is a transmembrane protein belonging to the ferlin protein family and is involved in glutamate transmitter release at the ribbon synapse of inner hair cells in the cochlea. The abnormal transmitter release at the synapse leads to impairment in activation of the cochlear nerve. Figure 9.1 shows audiological and vestibular findings in a 2-year-old girl with *OTOF* mutations. She showed severe hearing loss and preserved DPOAE, but ABRs were absent in both ears, indicating an auditory neuropathy (Fig. 9.1). She showed normal per-rotatory nystagmus in rotation tests and normal cVEMP responses in both ears, suggesting preserved vestibular function. Although there have been no reports on vestibular function in patients with OTOF mutations, patients with this mutation may have vestibular disorders. It has been shown that otoferlin is essential for calcium-dependent exocytosis in ribbon synapses at vestibular hair cells as well as at auditory hair cells [10].

9.3   Vestibular Involvement in Other Neuropathic Diseases

Involvements of vestibular nerve in other neuropathic diseases have been reported in various neuropathic diseases (Table 9.1).

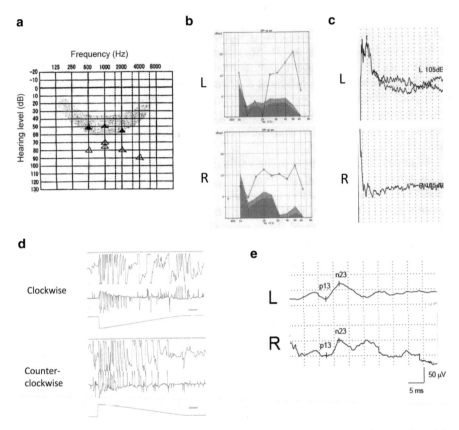

Fig. 9.1 Audiological and vestibular findings in a 2-year-old girl with *OTOF* mutation. (**a**) Audiogram. (**b**) Distortion product otoacoustic emission. (**c**) Auditory brainstem responses in response to 105 dBnHL clicks. (**d**) Results of dumped rotation test. (**e**) Cervical vestibular evoked myogenic potentials in response to 135 dBSPL tone bursts (5 ms). *L* left, *R* right

Table 9.1 Vestibular involvement in other neuropathic diseases

Etiology	Disease	Reference
Genetic mutation	Charcot-Marie-Tooth (CMT) disease	[12, 13]
	Dominant optic atrophy (DOA)	[15]
Autoimmune disorder	Guillain-Barre syndrome	[17]
	Chronic inflammatory demyelination polyneuropathy (CIDP)	[20]
Inflammation	Sarcoidosis	[22, 23]
Mitochondrial mutation	Friedreich's ataxia	[24, 25]
	Mitochondrial encephalomyopathy	[27]
Metabolic	Wernicke's encephalopathy	[30, 31]
	Diabetes mellitus	[32, 33]

9.3.1 Charcot-Marie-Tooth (CMT) Disease

CMT is a group of various inherited disorders of the peripheral nervous system characterized by progressive loss of muscle tissue and touch sensation in various parts of the body [11]. Patients with CMT have been clinically divided into two categories on the basis of nerve conduction velocity (NCV): slow conduction (CMT1) and normal conduction (CMT2). CMT is caused by mutations in neuronal proteins found in the myelin sheath and axon. The most common cause of CMT is the duplication of a large region on the short arm of chromosome 17 including the gene *PMP22*.

Jen et al. [12] reported that two patients with a point mutation in the PMP22 gene had a combination of vestibular dysfunction and peripheral neuropathy [12]. Poretti et al. [13] performed two kinds of vestibular function tests, the cVEMP test and the head impulse test which assesses the high-acceleration vestibuloocular reflex of the semicircular canals, in 15 CMT patients. They reported that the cVEMPs and head impulse tests were impaired in 75 % and 60 % of the patients, respectively, suggesting that the neuropathic processes of CMT frequently involve the vestibular nerve [13].

9.3.2 Dominant Optic Atrophy (DOA)

DOA is among the most common inherited optic neuropathy, characterized by progressive bilateral visual loss in childhood [14]. Retinal ganglion cell degeneration, affecting the small fibers of the papillomacular bundle, is characteristic of DOA. About 70 % of patients with DOA have pathogenic mutations in the nuclear gene (*OPA1*) encoding for the OPA1 protein. The most common extraocular manifestation in DOA is hearing loss in the form of auditory neuropathy [14].

Mizutari et al. [15] reported a patient with a mutation in OPA1 who had absent caloric responses in both ears and absent cVEMPs in one ear [15]. Santarelli et al. [14] reported that two of the nine patients with the OPA-1 missense mutation reported vertigo [14]. These patients might have had vestibular neuropathy as well as auditory neuropathy.

9.3.3 Guillain-Barre Syndrome (GBS)

GBS is a potentially life-threatening postinfectious neuropathy characterized by rapidly progressive, symmetrical weakness of the extremities [16]. About 25 % of patients develop respiratory dysfunction, and most patients show signs of autonomic dysfunction. The pathogenesis of GBS is considered to be caused by cross-reactive antibodies against gangliosides generated by molecular mimicry of pathogen-borne antigens. Diagnosis can usually be made from the clinical symptoms: progressive weakness in legs and arms and areflexia in weak limbs, which continue to progress for up to 4 weeks. Lumbar puncture shows increased numbers of mononuclear or polymorphonuclear cells in the cerebrospinal fluid.

Jacot and Weiner-Vacher [17] reported a patient with GBS who showed normal caloric responses but increased latencies in cVEMP responses, suggesting decreased conduction velocity in the central vestibulospinal pathways [17].

9.3.4 Chronic Inflammatory Demyelination Neuropathy (CIDP)

CIDP is defined by symmetric proximal and distal weakness with sensory signs and symptoms in both arms and legs in the presence of electrophysiological features consistent with demyelinating neuropathy. The symptoms of CIDP show a progressive course in 62 %, relapsing-remitting course in 26 %, and monophasic course in 12 % of patients [18]. The pathogenesis of CIDP is still unclear, but an autoimmune etiology is presumed because of the similarity of CIDP to experimental autoimmune neuritis in rats [19].

CIDP is frequently associated with cranial neuropathies. Frohman et al. [20] reported a patient with CIDP who had oscillopsia, disequilibrium, and gait disturbance [20]. Bilateral vestibulopathy of this patient was demonstrated by bithermal caloric tests, rotatory chair testing, and dynamic posturography. An MRI with gadolinium revealed enhancement of eight cranial nerves bilaterally. This patient's gait disturbance and vestibulopathy were improved by immunotherapy, suggesting immune-mediated vestibulopathy.

9.3.5 Sarcoidosis

Sarcoidosis is a systemic granulomatous disease whose origin is still unknown [21]. The typical histopathologic feature of sarcoidosis is a granuloma composed of epithelioid cells surrounded by mature lymphocytes and Langerhans-type and foreign-body-type giant cells. Respiratory symptoms are most common, but other symptoms such as general fatigue, dry eyes, or skin lesions are also frequent.

Neurologic involvement occurs in about 5 % of patients with sarcoidosis, in which the facial nerve is most frequently involved. The eighth nerve is the fourth most commonly affected nerve in neurosarcoidosis. Babin et al. [22] reported a patient with neurosarcoidosis in which the cochlear, vestibular, and facial nerves were involved. Histopathological examination of the temporal bone revealed degeneration of the labyrinthine neuroepithelium [22]. Agari et al. [23] reported a patient with neurosarcoidosis with hearing loss and unsteady gait [23]. The patient showed moderate sensorineural hearing loss and absent caloric responses in both ears.

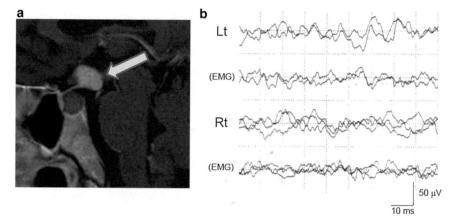

Fig. 9.2 Brain MRI and cVEMP responses in a 57-year-old man with neurosarcoidosis. This patient was referred to our clinic with a chief complaint of dizziness and instability while walking. (**a**) MRI of the brain. Neurosarcoidosis in the hypothalamus (*arrow*). (**b**) cVEMPs in response to 135 dB SPL tone burst showed no responses on both sides. *EMG* indicates background EMG (rectified). He showed no caloric nystagmus in both ears. *Lt* left, *Rt* right

Her hearing loss and vestibular dysfunction were significantly improved by administration of corticosteroids. Figure 9.2 shows results from a patient with neurosarcoidosis with bilateral involvement of the vestibular nerve.

9.3.6 Friedreich's Ataxia (FRDA)

FRDA is the most common autosomal recessive hereditary ataxic disease, which affects the central and peripheral nervous systems, heart, skeleton, and pancreas. FRDA is caused by a mutation in a homozygous guanine-adenine-adenine (GAA) trinucleotide repeat expansion on chromosome 9q13 which leads to a transcriptional defect of the frataxin gene. Deficiency of frataxin, a small mitochondrial protein, is responsible for all manifestations of FRDA. Clinically, ataxia of gait is almost always the initial manifestation of FRDA. Subsequently, involvement of the upper and lower limbs, dysarthria, and loss of sensation occurs.

Vestibular dysfunction is common in FRDA. Spoendlin [24] reported two sisters with FRDA who showed no caloric responses. Examination of the temporal bone revealed degeneration of the cochlear nerve and the ampullary branch of the vestibular nerve [24]. Fahey et al. [28] examined vestibular function in 20 FRDA patients using the head impulse test which measures high-frequency components of the vestibuloocular reflex and showed significantly reduced gain in both ears compared to controls [25].

9.3.7   Mitochondrial Encephalomyopathy

Mutations in mitochondrial DNA have a close association with sensorineural hearing loss [26]. Deafness is observed in about 70 % of patients with mitochondrial syndromes such as Kearns-Sayre syndrome, myoclonus epilepsy associated with ragged-red fibers, and mitochondrial encephalomyopathy, lactic acidosis, and stroke-like episodes (MELAS). Iwasaki et al. [27] performed caloric tests and cVEMPs in 13 patients with mitochondrial A3243G mutations and showed that most of those patients had bilateral vestibular dysfunction (10 of 13 showed abnormal caloric responses; 12 of 13 showed abnormal cVEMPs), suggesting that vestibular dysfunction is common in patients with mitochondrial encephalomyopathy [27]. However, results of galvanic cVEMPs, a test of retrolabyrinthine vestibular function, suggested that a labyrinthine lesion, not a retrolabyrinthine lesion, is responsible for vestibular dysfunction in these patients.

9.3.8   Wernicke's Encephalopathy

Wernicke's encephalopathy is an acute neuropsychiatric disorder resulting from deficiency in vitamin B1 (thiamine), which is associated with significant morbidity and mortality [28]. It is characterized by gaze-evoked nystagmus, ophthalmoplegia, mental status changes, and unsteadiness of stance and gait, although only 16 % of patients manifest all of these symptoms. The presumptive diagnosis of Wernicke's encephalopathy can be made by clinical symptoms and measurement of blood thiamine concentrations, but brain MRI is currently considered as the most valuable method to confirm a diagnosis. MRI studies typically show an increased T2 signal bilaterally and symmetrically in the paraventricular regions of the thalamus, hypothalamus, floor of the fourth ventricle, and midline cerebellum [29].

Furman and Becker [30] reported two patients with Wernicke's encephalopathy who showed hypoactive vestibular responses to both caloric and rotational stimuli. Both patients showed improved vestibular function following treatment with thiamine [30]. Choi et al. [31] performed head impulse tests in two patients with Wernicke's encephalopathy and reported selective involvement of the horizontal semicircular canals, sparing function in the anterior and posterior semicircular canals [31]. They suggested that this result might be due to selective vulnerability of neurons in the medial vestibular nucleus.

9.3.9   Diabetes Mellitus (DM)

DM is a metabolic disorder which causes hyperglycemia due to a lack of, or insensitivity to, insulin. Peripheral neuropathy is a major consequence of DM with up to 50 % of patients showing clinically significant neural injury during the disease course.

Several studies have demonstrated vestibular dysfunction in patient with DM on the basis of caloric responses [32, 33]. Klagenberg et al. [33] reported vestibular dysfunction in 60 % of patients with type 1 DM [33], suggesting peripheral involvement in the disease. On the other hand, Gawron et al. reported central vestibular involvement in patients with type I DM based on the results of electronystagmographic tests [32].

9.4 Idiopathic Bilateral Vestibulopathy (IBV)

IBV, which was first reported by Baloh and his colleagues in 1989 [34], is defined as an acquired bilateral vestibular dysfunction of unknown cause. Patients with IBV show absent or markedly decreased responses of the lateral semicircular canals as revealed by caloric and/or rotational tests. Their main clinical symptom is persistent imbalance, particularly in darkness, not accompanied by hearing loss or other neurologic dysfunctions. There are two types of IBV, sequential or progressive, according to their clinical courses.

Patients with sequential-type IBV show recurrent episodes of vertigo or dizziness. Initially, the unilateral vestibular end organs might be involved unilaterally, while later involvement of the contralateral side of the vestibular organs might produce symptoms and signs of bilateral vestibular loss. The possible etiology of the sequential type includes viral, ischemic, and autoimmune causes.

The other type of IBV is the progressive type. Patients of this type show a gradually progressive imbalance without episodic vertigo. Possible causes include inherited, toxic, and metabolic causes. IBV in some patients with this type may be caused by progressive degeneration of vestibular neurons.

By definition, IBV is diagnosed by absent or markedly decreased responses of the lateral semicircular canals. It is possible that other vestibular end organs, such as the utricle or the saccule, may be involved in IBV patients. To evaluate the involvement of the otolith organs in IBV, we recorded cVEMPs, which reflect the function of the saccule and its afferents, and ocular VEMPs (oVEMPs), which reflect the function of the utricle and its afferents, in 28 patients with IBV (19 men and 9 women, 36–80 years old).

All the patients had absent or markedly reduced caloric responses bilaterally. Figure 9.3 summarizes the results. For cVEMPs, 45 % of the patients showed bilaterally abnormal responses, 25 % showed unilaterally abnormal responses, and the remaining 30 % showed normal responses. For oVEMPs, 36 % showed bilaterally abnormal responses, 18 % showed unilaterally abnormal responses, and the remaining 46 % showed normal responses.

We classified these IBV patients into four groups according to the results of cVEMP and oVEMP testings (Table 9.2): those in which both oVEMPs and cVEMPs were abnormal (39 %), cVEMPs with normal oVEMPs (32 %), abnormal oVEMPs with normal cVEMPs (14 %), and both oVEMPs and cVEMPs normal (14 %).

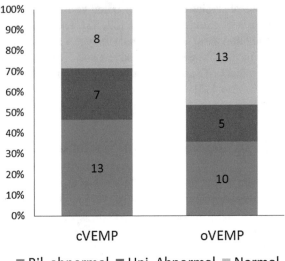

Fig. 9.3 Results of cVEMPs and oVEMPs in 28 patients with idiopathic bilateral vestibulopathy. *Bil. abnormal* bilaterally abnormal, *Uni. abnormal* unilaterally abnormal

Table 9.2 Result of cVEMPs and oVEMPs in 28 IBV patients

		cVEMP	
		Abnormal	Normal
oVEMP	Abnormal	11 (39 %)	4 (14 %)
	Normal	9 (32 %)	4 (14 %)

cVEMPs cervical vestibular evoked myogenic potentials, *oVEMPs* ocular vestibular evoked myogenic potentials

We compared postural stability by stabilometry in those IBV patients classified according to the results of the cVEMP and oVEMP tests (Fig. 9.4). Both the velocity of the movement and the envelopment area in the patient group with abnormal responses in both cVEMPs and oVEMPs were much worse than the other groups. The patients who had abnormal cVEMPs only or abnormal oVEMPs only had a tendency to show greater movement while standing as compared to normal groups, suggesting that the involvement of the otolith organs affects postural stability in patients with IBV.

Galvanic cVEMP testing is a form of cVEMP testing that is evoked by galvanic vestibular stimulation. Since galvanic vestibular stimulation directly activates retrolabyrinthine vestibular afferents, galvanic cVEMPs can discriminate between labyrinthine and retrolabyrinthine vestibular dysfunction when cVEMPs to air-conducted sound are absent. Fujimoto et al. [35] recorded galvanic cVEMPs in a patient with IBV. In this patient, both cVEMPs to ACS and galvanic cVEMPs were absent on the left side, suggesting that his vestibular lesions on the left side were retrolabyrinthine in origin [35].

Fig. 9.4 Results of
stabilometry in 28 patients
with idiopathic bilateral
vestibulopathy. (**a**) Velocity
of the center of pressure
(COP) with eyes closed.
(**b**) Envelopment area of
COP with eyes closed.
cVEMP + oVEMP:
patients who showed
abnormal cVEMP and
abnormal oVEMP.
cVEMP: patients who
showed abnormal cVEMP
and normal oVEMP.
oVEMP: patients who
showed normal cVEMP
and abnormal
oVEMP. Normal: patients
who showed normal
cVEMP and normal
oVEMP

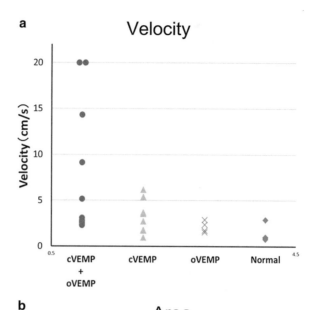

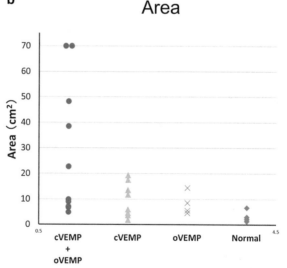

9.5 Summary

It is likely that many patients with auditory neuropathy as well as those with other
neuropathies have bilateral vestibular dysfunction. A proportion of IBV patients
appear to have retrolabyrinthine vestibular neuropathies. Since most patients with
bilateral involvement of the vestibular nerves do not have vestibular symptoms, it is
useful to perform vestibular function tests in patients with non-vestibular neuropathies in order to determine whether there is vestibular nerve involvement.

Developments of new vestibular function tests which can discriminate retrolabyrinthine lesions from labyrinthine lesions are necessary to correctly diagnose "vestibular neuropathy."

References

1. Starr A, Picton TW, Sininger Y, Hood LJ, Berlin CI. Auditory neuropathy. Brain. 1996;119(Pt 3):741–53.
2. Kaga K, Nakamura M, Shinogami M, Tsuzuku T, Yamada K, Shindo M. Auditory nerve disease of both ears revealed by auditory brainstem responses, electrocochleography and otoacoustic emissions. Scand Audiol. 1996;25(4):233–8.
3. Rance G, Starr A. Pathophysiological mechanisms and functional hearing consequences of auditory neuropathy. Brain. 2015;138(Pt 11):3141–58. doi:10.1093/brain/awv270.
4. Fujikawa S, Starr A. Vestibular neuropathy accompanying auditory and peripheral neuropathies. Arch Otolaryngol Head Neck Surg. 2000;126(12):1453–6.
5. Masuda T, Kaga K. Influence of aging over 10 years on auditory and vestibular functions in three patients with auditory neuropathy. Acta Otolaryngol. 2011;131(5):562–8. doi:10.3109/00016489.2010.534112.
6. Sazgar AA, Yazdani N, Rezazadeh N, Yazdi AK. Vestibular evoked myogenic potential (VEMP) in patients with auditory neuropathy: auditory neuropathy or audiovestibular neuropathy? Acta Otolaryngol. 2010;130(10):1130–4. doi:10.3109/00016481003727582.
7. Sheykholeslami K, Kaga K, Murofushi T, Hughes DW. Vestibular function in auditory neuropathy. Acta Otolaryngol. 2000;120(7):849–54.
8. Starr A, Michalewski HJ, Zeng FG, Fujikawa-Brooks S, Linthicum F, Kim CS, et al. Pathology and physiology of auditory neuropathy with a novel mutation in the MPZ gene (Tyr145->Ser). Brain. 2003;126(Pt 7):1604–19. doi:10.1093/brain/awg156.
9. Rodriguez-Ballesteros M, del Castillo FJ, Martin Y, Moreno-Pelayo MA, Morera C, Prieto F, et al. Auditory neuropathy in patients carrying mutations in the otoferlin gene (OTOF). Hum Mutat. 2003;22(6):451–6. doi:10.1002/humu.10274.
10. Dulon D, Safieddine S, Jones SM, Petit C. Otoferlin is critical for a highly sensitive and linear calcium-dependent exocytosis at vestibular hair cell ribbon synapses. J Neurosci. 2009;29(34):10474–87. doi:10.1523/jneurosci.1009-09.2009.
11. Krajewski KM, Lewis RA, Fuerst DR, Turansky C, Hinderer SR, Garbern J, et al. Neurological dysfunction and axonal degeneration in Charcot-Marie-Tooth disease type 1A. Brain. 2000;123(Pt 7):1516–27.
12. Jen J, Baloh RH, Ishiyama A, Baloh RW. Dejerine-Sottas syndrome and vestibular loss due to a point mutation in the PMP22 gene. J Neurol Sci. 2005;237(1–2):21–4. doi:10.1016/j.jns.2005.05.003.
13. Poretti A, Palla A, Tarnutzer AA, Petersen JA, Weber KP, Straumann D, et al. Vestibular impairment in patients with Charcot-Marie-tooth disease. Neurology. 2013;80(23):2099–105. doi:10.1212/WNL.0b013e318295d72a.
14. Santarelli R, Rossi R, Scimemi P, Cama E, Valentino ML, La Morgia C, et al. OPA1-related auditory neuropathy: site of lesion and outcome of cochlear implantation. Brain. 2015;138(Pt 3):563–76. doi:10.1093/brain/awu378.
15. Mizutari K, Matsunaga T, Inoue Y, Kaneko H, Yagi H, Namba K, et al. Vestibular dysfunction in a Japanese patient with a mutation in the gene OPA1. J Neurol Sci. 2010;293(1–2):23–8. doi:10.1016/j.jns.2010.03.014.
16. van den Berg B, Walgaard C, Drenthen J, Fokke C, Jacobs BC, van Doorn PA. Guillain-Barre syndrome: pathogenesis, diagnosis, treatment and prognosis. Nat Rev Neurol. 2014;10(8):469–82. doi:10.1038/nrneurol.2014.121.

17. Jacot E, Wiener-Vacher S. Potential value of vestibular evoked myogenic potentials in paediatric neuropathies. J Vestib Res. 2008;18(4):231–7.
18. Eftimov F, van Schaik I. Chronic inflammatory demyelinating polyradiculoneuropathy: update on clinical features, phenotypes and treatment options. Curr Opin Neurol. 2013;26(5):496–502. doi:10.1097/WCO.0b013e328363bfa4.
19. Hughes RA, Allen D, Makowska A, Gregson NA. Pathogenesis of chronic inflammatory demyelinating polyradiculoneuropathy. J Peripher Nerv Syst. 2006;11(1):30–46. doi:10.1111/j.1085-9489.2006.00061.x.
20. Frohman EM, Tusa R, Mark AS, Cornblath DR. Vestibular dysfunction in chronic inflammatory demyelinating polyneuropathy. Ann Neurol. 1996;39(4):529–35. doi:10.1002/ana.410390415.
21. Dempsey OJ, Paterson EW, Kerr KM, Denison AR. Sarcoidosis BMJ. 2009;339:b3206. doi:10.1136/bmj.b3206.
22. Babin RW, Liu C, Aschenbrener C. Histopathology of neurosensory deafness in sarcoidosis. Ann Otol Rhinol Laryngol. 1984;93(4 Pt 1):389–93.
23. Agari D, Koide R, Kashiyama T, Yoshida H, Naito R, Bandoh M. Neurosarcoidosis: a treatable cause of vestibular dysfunction. Lancet. 2007;369(9564):878. doi:10.1016/s0140-6736(07)60417-6.
24. Spoendlin H. Optic cochleovestibular degenerations in hereditary ataxias. II. Temporal bone pathology in two cases of Friedreich's ataxia with vestibulo-cochlear disorders. Brain. 1974;97(1):41–8.
25. Fahey MC, Cremer PD, Aw ST, Millist L, Todd MJ, White OB, et al. Vestibular, saccadic and fixation abnormalities in genetically confirmed Friedreich ataxia. Brain. 2008;131(Pt 4):1035–45. doi:10.1093/brain/awm323.
26. Wallace DC. Diseases of the mitochondrial DNA. Annu Rev Biochem. 1992;61:1175–212. doi:10.1146/annurev.bi.61.070192.005523.
27. Iwasaki S, Egami N, Fujimoto C, Chihara Y, Ushio M, Kashio A, et al. The mitochondrial A3243G mutation involves the peripheral vestibule as well as the cochlea. Laryngoscope. 2011;121(8):1821–4. doi:10.1002/lary.21879.
28. Sechi G, Serra A. Wernicke's encephalopathy: new clinical settings and recent advances in diagnosis and management. Lancet Neurol. 2007;6(5):442–55. doi:10.1016/s1474-4422(07)70104-7.
29. Antunez E, Estruch R, Cardenal C, Nicolas JM, Fernandez-Sola J, Urbano-Marquez A. Usefulness of CT and MR imaging in the diagnosis of acute Wernicke's encephalopathy. AJR Am J Roentgenol. 1998;171(4):1131–7. doi:10.2214/ajr.171.4.9763009.
30. Furman JM, Becker JT. Vestibular responses in Wernicke's encephalopathy. Ann Neurol. 1989;26(5):669–74. doi:10.1002/ana.410260513.
31. Choi KD, Oh SY, Kim HJ, Kim JS. The vestibulo-ocular reflexes during head impulse in Wernicke's encephalopathy. J Neurol Neurosurg Psychiatry. 2007;78(10):1161–2. doi:10.1136/jnnp.2007.121061.
32. Gawron W, Pospiech L, Orendorz-Fraczkowska K, Noczynska A. Are there any disturbances in vestibular organ of children and young adults with type I diabetes? Diabetologia. 2002;45(5):728–34. doi:10.1007/s00125-002-0813-x.
33. Klagenberg KF, Zeigelboim BS, Jurkiewicz AL, Martins-Bassetto J. Vestibulocochlear manifestations in patients with type I diabetes mellitus. Braz J Otorhinolaryngol. 2007;73(3):353–8.
34. Baloh RW, Jacobson K, Honrubia V. Idiopathic bilateral vestibulopathy. Neurology. 1989;39(2 Pt 1):272–5.
35. Fujimoto C, Iwasaki S, Matsuzaki M, Murofushi T. Lesion site in idiopathic bilateral vestibulopathy: a galvanic vestibular-evoked myogenic potential study. Acta Otolaryngol. 2005;125(4):430–2. doi:10.1080/00016480410024668.

Chapter 10
Vestibular Development of Children with Inner Ear Malformation and Cochlear Nerve Deficiency

Takeshi Masuda and Kimitaka Kaga

Abstract Motor development in children with inner ear malformation or cochlear nerve deficiency (CND) is often delayed. A reason for delayed head control and independent walking may be the loss of muscle from the vestibule, and, thus, sufficient tension cannot be maintained. A total of 12 children with bilateral inner ear malformation and 4 children with bilateral CND were studied. The development of head control and independent walking in all of the children with bilateral inner ear malformation and bilateral CND was delayed. For evaluation of vestibular function, a damped-rotational chair test was performed, and the horizontal nystagmus was recorded by using an electronystagmography (ENG). These 10 of 12 children with bilateral inner ear malformation and two of four children with bilateral CND showed reduced response to the rotational chair test at the initial time. The follow-up examination performed in all of the children with bilateral inner ear malformation whose vestibular function appeared was compared with the initial examination. The development of motor function in children with bilateral inner ear malformation and CND is related with not only central compensation but also vestibular development.

Keywords Rotation test • Electronystagmography • Nystagmus

T. Masuda (✉)
Department of Otolaryngology, Head & Neck Surgery, Nihon University School of Medicine, 30-1 Oyaguchi-Kamicho, Itabashik-ku, Tokyo 173-8610, Japan
e-mail: masusam@nifty.cm

K. Kaga
National Institute of Sensory Organs, National Tokyo Medical Center, 2 5 1 Higashigaoka, Meguro-Ku, Tokyo 152-8902, Japan

Center for Speech and Hearing Disorders, International University of Health and Welfare Clinic, 2600-6 Kitakanemaru, Ohtawara, Tochigi 324-0011, Japan

© Springer Science+Business Media Singapore 2017
K. Kaga (ed.), *Cochlear Implantation in Children with Inner Ear Malformation and Cochlear Nerve Deficiency*, Modern Otology and Neurotology, DOI 10.1007/978-981-10-1400-0_10

10.1   Introduction

The developmental neurology of balance impairment in infants and children began from the observation of postural reflex of infants and children. Kaga in 1980 examined the vestibuloocular reflex (VOR) quantitatively in children with severe hearing loss using a rotational chair and demonstrated that head control and independent walking are delayed when the VOR is lacking [1]. Currently, inner ear morphology can be observed in detail due to the development of high-resolution CT, and inner ear malformations and narrowing of the internal auditory canal can be revealed. However, there have been no reports that follow up on changes of the VOR due to development. Therefore, we evaluated the vestibular function of children with bilateral severe hearing loss using a rotational chair test. In addition, we performed a follow-up study on the relationship between vestibular function and motor development for which head control and independent walking were used as indicators of motor development.

10.2   Material and Methods

10.2.1   Patients

Twelve children with a bilateral inner ear malformation and four children with a bilateral cochlear nerve deficiency (CND) who visited the Tokyo Medical Center Hospital for infants and children with hearing loss and language disorder clinic. None of the children had cochlear implant surgery prior to the initial examination. Inner ear malformations were classified according to the classification by Sennaroglu et al. [2].

10.2.2   Motor Development

Head control (the state that a motion of the head is controllable by itself) and independent walking (the state that no support is needed when walking) were used as indicators of motor development. Based on the results of an infant and children physical development survey report in 2010 conducted by the Ministry of Health, Labour and Welfare of Japan, a delay in motor development was determined when head control was later than 5 months and independent walking was later than 14 months, which are the 97th percentile values.

10.2.3   Damped-Rotational Chair Test

Earth-vertical axis rotation (EVAR) was used for the rotational chair test. A damped-rotational chair test similar to the protocol of Kaga [1] was performed using a computer-controlled rotational chair (Nagashima Co., Ltd., type S-II). For the safety of the children, a parent sat on the rotational chair first and then held the child on their lap during the rotational chair test. The test was performed in the dark in order to reduce the influence of the visual suppression, and the velocity was decelerated by 4° per second from the initial velocity of 160° per second. Right rotation was performed first, followed by left rotation after a 5-min interval. Nystagmus was recorded by electronystagmography (ENG). The electrodes were placed near the lateral canthus of both eyes to record the eye movement in the horizontal direction. The number of beats of nystagmus during rotation and duration of time for nystagmus was measured, and the average values of the left and right rotations were obtained. When both were less than 50 % of the age control data of Kaga [1], the vestibular function was determined to be reduced.

10.3   Result

10.3.1   Inner Ear Malformation

All 12 children showed delayed motor development, especially independent walking. The response of damped-rotational chair test is reduced in 11 of 12 children at the first time. The follow-up examination of the 12 children with inner ear malformation showed that distinct nystagmus began to appear compared to the initial examination in 11 children who showed reduced nystagmus at the first examination (Table 10.1).

10.3.2   Cochlear Nerve Deficiency

All four children showed delayed motor development. The response of damped-rotational chair test is reduced in two of four children (Table 10.2).

10.4   Discussion

Motor development in children with bilateral inner ear malformation is often delayed. A reason for delayed head control and independent walking may be due to the loss of muscle from the vestibule, and, thus, sufficient tension cannot be

Table 10.1 Results of motor development and nystagmus during rotation of children who had a bilateral inner ear malformation

No.	Age	Type of the cochlear anomaly	Type of the vestibular anomaly	Time duration (s)	Number of beats	Head control	Independent walking
1	2 years 6 months	Bilateral common cavity	Bilateral common cavity	3.5	3.5	4 months	1 year 6 months
	3 years 5 months			0	0		
	4 years 9 months			39	28		
2	3 years 3 months	Bilateral IP-I	Bilateral dysplasia	6	3.5	4 months	2 years 4 months
	5 years 7 months			37	22		
3	6 months	Bilateral common cavity	Bilateral common cavity	0	0	4 months	1 year 6 months
	4 years 7 months			31.	28.5		
	6 years 5 months			36	43.5		
4	9 months	Bilateral IP-II	Bilateral dysplasia	0	0	9 months	1 year 6 months
	1 year 10 months			37	40.5		
5	1 year 7 months	Lt. IP-I	Lt. dysplasia	12.5	8	6 months	2 years 0 month
	3 years 2 months	Rt. Michel	Rt. Michel	2.5	3.5		
	5 years 1 month			16.5	19.5		
6	6 months	Bilateral IP-II	Bilateral Hypoplasia	0	0	6 months	2 years 0 month
	1 year 4 months			0	0		
	1 year 11 months			0	0		
	3 years 2 months			2	2		
	4 years 2 months			28	18.5		
7	2 years 3 months	Lt. IP-I	Lt. dysplasia	0	0	6 months	2 years 0 month
	3 years 8 months	Rt. hypoplasia	Rt. hypoplasia	29.5	34		
	4 years 7 months			35.5	48.5		
8	9 months	Lt. IP-II	Bilateral dysplasia	0	0	6 months	1 year 2 months
	1 year 2 months	Rt. IP-I		9.5	11		
	2 years 0 month			28	21		

(continued)

Table 10.1 (continued)

No.	Age	Type of the cochlear anomaly	Type of the vestibular anomaly	Time duration (s)	Number of beats	Head control	Independent walking
9	1 year 10 months	Bilateral common cavity	Bilateral common cavity	5	6	6 months	1 year 6 months
	4 years 9 months			33	38		
10	5 months	Bilateral common cavity	Bilateral common cavity	28	30	7 months	1 year 3 months
	1 year 5 months			8	8.5		
	2 years 3 months			23.5	24.5		
11	1 year 5 months	Bilateral IP-II	Bilateral dysplasia	5	4	6 months	2 years 0 month
	1 year 8 months			25	12		
12	6 months	Bilateral common cavity	Bilateral common cavity	0	0	7 months	1 year 7 months
	1 year 0 month			15	10		
	1 year 2 months			15	12.5		
	1 year 7 months			18.5	18		

IP-I incomplete partition type I, *IP-II* incomplete partition type II [2]

Table 10.2 Results of motor development and nystagmus during rotation of children who had a bilateral CND

No.	Age	Time duration (s)	Number of beats	Head control	Independent walking
1	4 years 4 months	0	0	1 year, 4 months	4 years 4 months
2	2 years 2 months	10.5	9	6 months	1 year 10 months
	3 years 5 months	13	10		
3	5 years 2 months	37.5	31	10 months	2 years 4 months
4	1 year 2 months	19	22.5	6 months	–

Number of beats

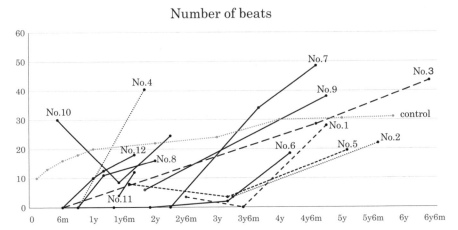

Fig. 10.1 The time course and the number of beats of nystagmus during rotation of all 12 children who had a bilateral inner ear malformation. The *dashed line* indicates control data by Kaga [1]

maintained [3]. In children with bilateral inner ear malformation or bilateral CND, not only hearing but also the vestibular nerve and vestibular sensory cells may have abnormalities that cause a delay in motor development [4]. This study also showed that motor development, such as head control and independent walking, was delayed in all children with bilateral inner ear malformation or bilateral CND. Nystagmus was more difficult to elicit in the younger age children in the caloric test, whereas it appeared regardless of age in the rotation test. As evidenced by a canal-plugging experiment in monkeys, the rotation test is one of the most stimulating tests among the vestibular function tests because it applies stimulus to the semicircular canals and otolith organs in both ears [5]. Therefore, it can detect the response even when the VOR is very weak.

Since 2008 in our facility, the damped-rotational chair test is performed, and the vestibular function, along with motor development, is evaluated before cochlear implant surgery. In the results, all of 12 children with bilateral inner ear malformation showed delayed motor development; also all of four children with bilateral CND showed delayed motor development.

Eleven of 12 children with bilateral inner ear malformation and two of four children with CND showed reduced response to the initial rotational chair test. The follow-up examination was carried out for all children with bilateral inner ear malformation. As a result, all children with bilateral inner ear malformation (100%) began to show a distinct VOR compared to the initial examination.

Figures 10.1, 10.2, 10.3, and 10.4 no. 1 child with bilateral common cavity deformity, first examination at the age of 2 years 6 months was no response. After

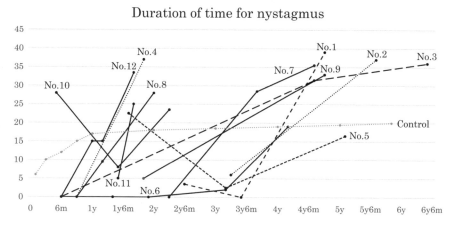

Fig. 10.2 The time course and the duration of time for nystagmus during rotation of all 12 children who had a bilateral inner ear malformation. The *dashed line* indicates control data by Kaga [2]

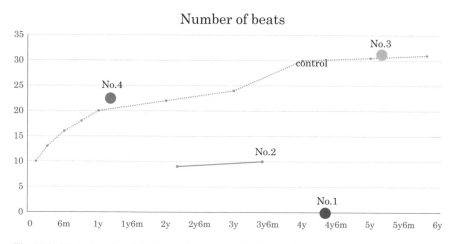

Fig. 10.3 Plotted results of the beats of nystagmus during rotation of all four children who had a CND. The *dashed line* indicates control data by Kaga [2]

2 years 3 months from first examination, at the age of 4 years 9 months who appeared VOR clearly (Figs. 10.5, 10.6, and 10.7).

CND no. 1 child was tested at the age of 4 years and 4 months, but has no response to the rotational chair test, because this child has severe CND (Figs. 10.8 and 10.9).

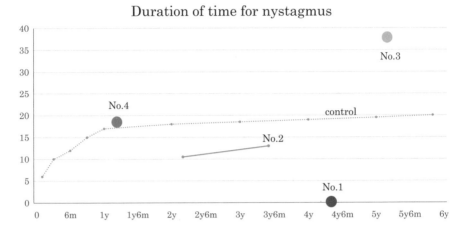

Fig. 10.4 Plotted results of the duration of time for nystagmus during rotation of all four children who had a CND. The *dashed line* indicates control data by Kaga [2]

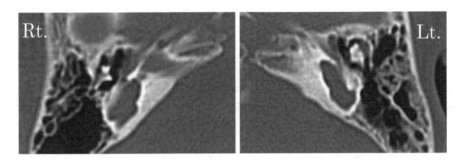

Fig. 10.5 CT imaging of common cavity deformity of no. 1 child

The reason why the VOR did not appear in the initial examination, but began to appear in the follow-up in this study. Taking from embryological knowledge, a membranous labyrinth is completed viviparously in 9 months. However, the vestibular sensory neuron is completed in 23 weeks time. Furthermore, the vestibular nerve is completed in 5 months. Although the form of a membranous labyrinth is in the state stopped in 6 weeks of viviparous time in common cavity malformation, after that myelinization of the vestibular nerve and maturation of the sensory cells embryologically [6, 7]. Figure 10.10 is drawn from embryological knowledge by Masuda et al. [8]. In regard to cases with the common cavity, malformations were

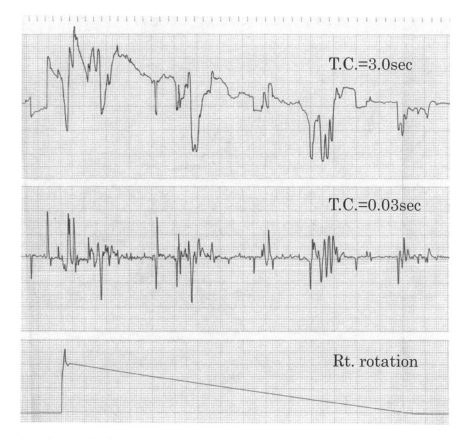

Fig. 10.6 Results of damped-rotation chair test at the age of 2 years and 6 months of no. 1 child

examined as an example. The appearance of the VOR with age in children with inner ear malformation may be due to the maturation of the vestibular nerve, maturation of the macula (vestibular sensory cells), or both (Fig. 10.10). In the case of CND, there exist two types of CND: one is a normal vestibular nerve, and the other is a vestibular nerve deficiency (Fig. 10.11).

Children with bilateral inner ear malformation or bilateral CND show a delay in motor development in their infancy but acquire vestibular compensation from the CNS or muscle tone due to the reflex from the vestibular labyrinth and growth. By junior high or high school, the children can perform most exercises without prob-

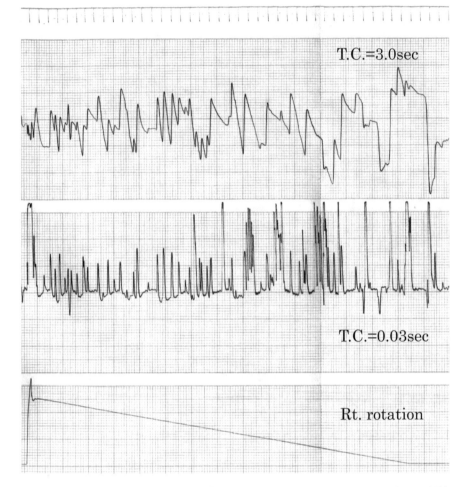

Fig. 10.7 Results of damped-rotation chair test at the age of 4 years and 9 months of no. 1 child. VOR appeared and was compared with the results at the age of 2 years and 6 months

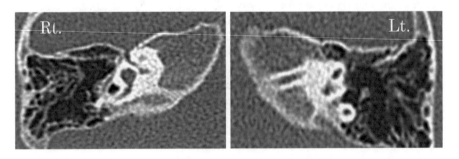

Fig. 10.8 CT imaging of CND no. 1 child who had severe CND

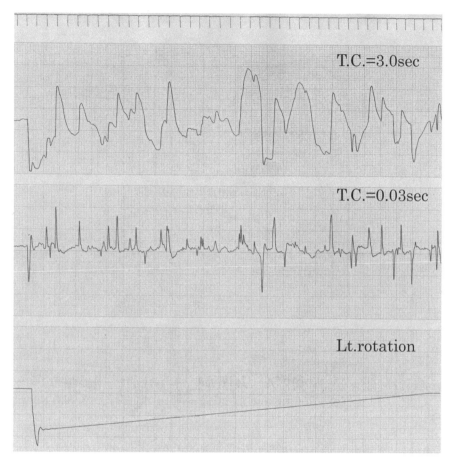

Fig. 10.9 Results of damped-rotation chair test at the age of 4 years and 4 months of no. 1 child. Direction of the rotation is left, but nystagmus-like eye movements appeared to the right. This eye movement is unrelated to VOR

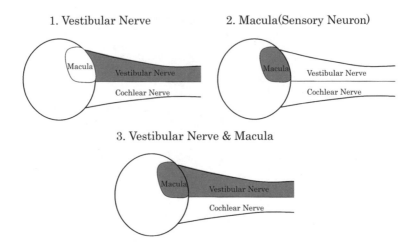

1. Vestibular Nerve   2. Macula(Sensory Neuron)

3. Vestibular Nerve & Macula

Fig. 10.10 Acquisition of the VOR in children with inner ear malformation [8]. (1) Development of the vestibular nerve. (2) Maturation of the macula (vestibular sensory cells). (3) Both 1 and 2

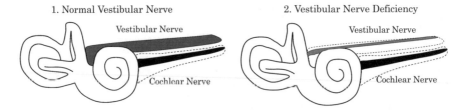

1. Normal Vestibular Nerve   2. Vestibular Nerve Deficiency

Fig. 10.11 The type of CND. (1) Normal vestibular nerve. (2) Vestibular nerve deficiency

lems [3]. This study reconfirmed that head control and independent walking are delayed if the acquisition of the VOR is insufficient. However, the VOR may be acquired with growth even if it is reduced during early childhood. It is necessary to accurately evaluate the vestibular function in children to determine the proper rehabilitation strategy [9].

References

1. Kaga K, Suzuki JI, Marsh RR, Tanaka Y. Influence of labyrinthine hypoactivity on gross motor development of infants. Ann N Y Acad Sci. 1981;374:412–20. doi:10.1111/j.1749-6632.1981. tb30887.x.
2. Sennaroglu L, Saatci I. A new classification for cochleovestibular malformations. Laryngoscope. 2002;112:2230–41. doi:10.1097/00005537-200212000-00019.
3. Kaga K. Vestibular compensation in infants and children with congenital and acquired vestibular loss in both ears. Int J Pediatr Otorhinolaryngol. 1999;49:215–24. doi:10.1016/ S0165-5876(99)00206-2.
4. Kaga K, Shinjo Y, Jin Y, Takegoshi H. Vestibular failure in children with congenital deafness. Int J Audiol. 2008;47:590–9. doi:10.1080/14992020802331222.
5. Cohen B, Suzuki JI, Raphan T. Role of the otolith organs in generation of horizontal nystagmus: effects of selective labyrinthine lesions. Brain Res. 1983;276:159–64. doi:10.1016/0006-8993(83)90558-9.
6. Moore KL, Persaud TVN, Torchia MG. Development of peripheral nervous system. The development human clinical oriented embryology. 9th ed. Philadelphia: Elsevier Saunders; 2012. p. 423–5.
7. Moore KL, Persaud TVN, Torchia MG. Development of ears. The development human clinical oriented embryology. 9th ed. Philadelphia: Elsevier Saunders; 2012. p. 441–9.
8. Masuda T, Kaga K. Relationship between acquisition of motor function and vestibular function in children with bilateral severe hearing loss. Acta Otolaryngol. 2014;134:672–8. doi:10.3109 /00016489.2014.890290.
9. Nandi R, Luxon LM. Development and assessment of the vestibular system. Int J Audiol. 2008;47:566–77. doi:10.1080/14992020802324540.

Chapter 11
Vestibular-Evoked Myogenic Potential After Cochlear Implantion

Kimitaka Kaga and Yulian Jin

Abstract Vestibular-evoked myogenic potential (VEMP) recording is a new tool for exploring the pathways from the sacculus, inferior vestibular nerve, and vestibular nucleus to sternocleidomastoid muscles (SCMs) in pediatric otology and neurotology. c-VEMP (saccular origin) and o-VEMP (utriculus origin) are clinically applied for a different diagnosis. After cochlear implantion, c-VEMPs are possible to record because of an electrical current spread from cochlear nerve which stimulates the inferior vestibular nerve.

Keywords VEMP • Sacculus • Utriculus • Vestibular development • Cochlear implantion

11.1 VEMPs of Normal Child Development

Although the muscle tone of neonates and young infants is poor compared with that of grown children and adults, it is possible to record VEMPs from the SCM during infancy and early childhood. Sheykholeslami et al. [1] reported that reproducible biphasic VEMPs are recorded from the SCM of all the infants they examined (12 healthy infants and children, aged 1–12 months) using loud and short-tone burst sounds. Typical developmental changes in VEMPs in infants and children are shown in Fig. 11.1 [2]. In these normal infants and children, air-conducted sound evoked a

K. Kaga (✉)
National Institute of Sensory Organs, National Tokyo Medical Center,
2-5-1 Higashigaoka, Meguro-Ku, Tokyo 152-8902, Japan

Center for Speech and Hearing Disorders, International University of Health
and Welfare Clinic, 2600-6 Kitakanemaru, Ohtawara, Tochigi 324-0011, Japan
e-mail: kaga@kankakuki.go.jp

Y. Jin
Department of Otorhinolaryngology, Yanbian University Hospital,
No. 1327, Juzi Street, Yanji 133 000, Republic of China

© Springer Science+Business Media Singapore 2017
K. Kaga (ed.), *Cochlear Implantation in Children with Inner Ear Malformation
and Cochlear Nerve Deficiency*, Modern Otology and Neurotology,
DOI 10.1007/978-981-10-1400-0_11

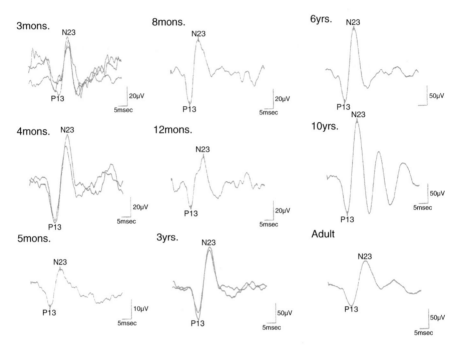

Fig. 11.1 Typical developmental changes in vestibular-evoked myogenic potentials (c-VMEPs) in normal infant and children

biphasic response (p13 and n23 peaks) of VEMPs that were of larger amplitude and shorter latency than those in adults. The difference in VEMPs on the side of the stimulated ear is due to developmental changes in the distance of the pathway between the sacculus and the SCM and changes in the strength of muscles. However, neonatal VEMPs varied in amplitude, with consistent timing for peak p13 but sorer n23 latencies than those in adult VEMPs.

11.2 VEMPs in Infants with Congenital Profound Hearing Loss

Colebatch et al. [3] showed that VEMPs were evident at a high incidence in patients with profound sensorineural hearing loss, but that they were abolished in all of their patients who underwent unilateral vestibular neurectomy. These authors also reported the VEMPs were abolished in some but not all patients with unilateral loss of a caloric response after vestibular neuritis. They hypothesized that VEMPs are of vestibular origin and that the saccule is probably an acoustically sensitive organ.

In our study, 67 % of the 54 ears of 33 children with congenital profound hearing loss showed normal VEMPs (Fig. 11.2), but 5 % of ears of the children showed abnormal VEMPs with low amplitude. This is a surprising finding because they cannot hear air-conducted loud click stimuli at all. However, they have VEMPs,

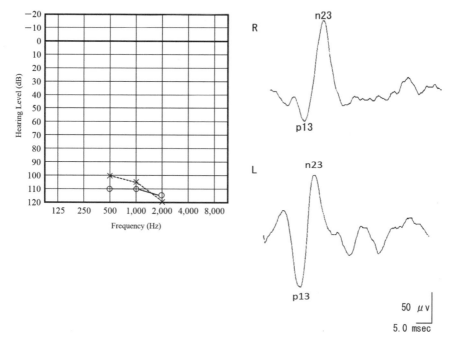

Fig. 11.2 Click-evoked normal VEMPs (*right*) and audiogram (*left*) of a child with congenital profound hearing loss

suggesting that VEMP testing can illuminate vestibular activity in deaf infants and children.

Sheykholeslami et al. [4, 5] confirmed that saccular origin of this short-latency acoustic response and that a saccular acoustic response persist in the human ear and has a well-defined frequency tuning curve. Currently, recorded VEMPs are induced using various stimuli including clicks [3], tone bursts [4], electrical stimuli [6], bone-conducted sounds [7], and head taps [8].

11.3 VEMPs in Children with No Inner Ear Malformation After Cochlear Implantation

The cochlear function of both ears is markedly impaired in infants and children who are candidates for cochlear implantation. However, vestibular function is also impaired in 10–20 % of such infants. After cochlear implantation, patients can hear speech sounds, which are converted to electrical signals in a speech processor; these signals are transmitted to the internal receiver under the scalp ad conducted to the electrodes in the cochlea. Thus, cochlea nerves that are stimulated electrically convey information to the central auditory brainstem pathway and auditory cortex.

There are two problems for vestibular end organs after cochlear implantation. One is traumatic damage of vestibular end organs incurred following insertion of

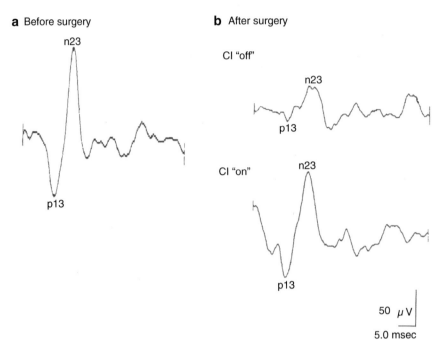

Fig. 11.3 Changes in VEMPs before and after cochlear implantation. (**a**) Before surgery. (**b**) Switched-off cochlear implant (*CI*) after surgery and switched-on CI after surgery

the electrodes of the cochlear implant into the scala tympani. Tien and Linthicum histopathologically analyzed the vestibular apparatus from human temporal bones after cochlear implantation was carried out [9]. The other problem is that electrical stimulation may spread not only the cochlear nerve but also the facial nerve or the vestibular nerve in patients with a multichannel cochlear implant because of current spread. Based on these findings, VEMPs are considered useful for evaluating electrical current spread to the inferior vestibular nerve.

Jin et al. compared VEMPs before and after surgery [10]. Before surgery, 6 of the 12 children showed normal VEMPs, 1 showed a decrease in the amplitude of VEMPs, and 5 showed no VEMPs. After surgery, with the cochlear implant switched off, 11 showed no VEMPs, and 1 showed decreased VEMPs. These results reveal that even normal VEMPS disappear owing to trauma following electrode insertion. With the cochlear implant switched on, four children showed normal VEMPs, but eight did not (Fig. 11.3). This can be explained by the fact that these four children's inferior vestibular nerves were stimulated by the spread of electrical current from the cochlear implant. We questioned why one-third of these children with cochlear implants showed VEMPs, but others did not. Later, Jin et al. demonstrated that VEMPs evoked by cochlear implants may be related to an electrical current intensity at a comfortable level (C level), particularly in channels that are closer to the apical turn of the cochlea [11].

The patients who showed no VEMPs with the cochlear implant switched on may require higher current intensities to elicit clear VEMPs (if they need to be recorded). However, it is difficult to increase current intensity in such children because they feel pain or facial nerve stimulation when the current intensity is higher than the C level.

11.4 VEMPs in Children with Inner Ear Malformation After Cochlear Implantation

Inner ear malformations and cochlear nerve deficiency (CND) present a major inner ear disorder in approximately 20 % of children with congenital sensorineural hearing loss [12]. They are usually characterized by profound hearing loss, and their development delays gross motor functions such as head control or independent walking, because such functions are related to abnormal inner ear structures [13]. However, it is not easy to unequivocally determine whether vestibular sensory cells of semicircular canals and otolith organs or primary vestibular afferent neurons are present in patients with inner ear malformations, particularly common cavity deformity. In an embryological study, it has been found that, in the human fetal developmental stage, the vestibular system develops earlier than the cochlear system [14]. Thus, it is speculated that sensory cells of vestibular end organs and vestibular afferent neurons may be present in patient with inner ear malformations, which is similar to early-stage inner ear development.

In our study, we reported that VEMPs could be elicited with the cochlear implant switched on and suggested that the electrical stimulation of a cochlear implant may directly stimulate the inferior vestibular nerve [10, 11]. If VEMPs are evoked with the cochlear implant switched on, it suggests that some of the inferior vestibular neurons are present. In contrast, if VEMPs are absent with the cochlear implant switched on, it suggests that the inferior vestibular neurons may be absent.

Seven children with inner ear malformation and CND who underwent cochlear implantation participated in this study (Table 11.1). The patients had common cav-

Table 11.1 Profiles of patients

Patient no.	Ear	Age at surgery (years)	Type of inner ear malformation	CI type	Speech processor	Strategy	Pulse width	VEMP after CI	
								CI off	CI on
1	L	5	Common cavity	24M	ESPrit 3G	ACE	25	+	+
2	R	5	IP-II LVAS	24M	Sprint	ACE	25	−	+
3	R	4	IP-I, narrow IAC	24R	Sprint	SPEAK	200	−	+
4	L	3	Common cavity	24M	Sprint	SPEAK	50	−	+
5	R	3	IP-I	22M	ESPrit 3G	SPEAK	0	−	+
6	R	4	IP-I	24M	Sprint	ACE	25	−	+
7	L	2	CND	24M	Sprint	ACE	100	−	+

IP-I incomplete partition type I, *IP-II* incomplete partition type II, *IAC* internal auditory canal, *LVAS* large vestibular aqueduct syndrome, *CI* cochlear implantation, *CND* cochlear nerve deficiency

ity deformity ($n = 2$), incomplete partition type I ($n = 2$), incomplete partition type II ($n = 1$), and CND. After surgery, VEMPs were recorded with the cochlear implant device switched both off and on. All the patients showed VEMPs with the cochlear implant switched on (Figs. 11.4 and 11.5).

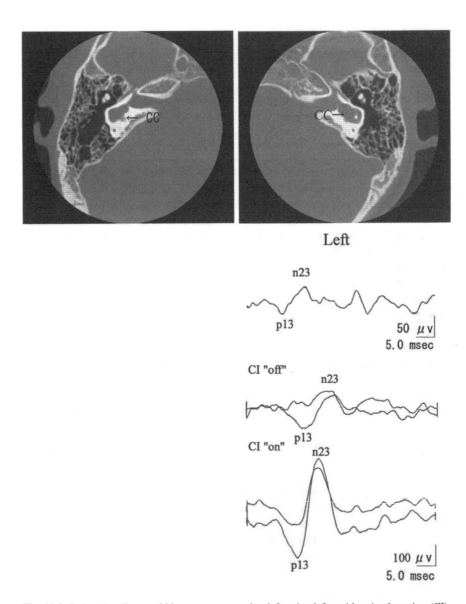

Fig. 11.4 Patient 1: a 7-year-old boy, common cavity deformity, left cochlear implantation (CI). CT scan demonstrated a deformity of the common cavity communicating with IAC. VEMPs were present with the CI on [10, 11]

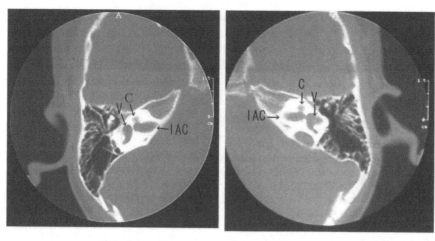

Right

CI "off"

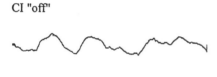

CI "on"

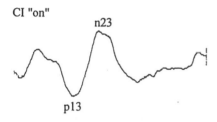

Fig. 11.5 Patient 5: an 8-year-old boy, IP-I deformity, right CT. CT scan demonstrated IP-I deformity. After CI, VEMPs were present with the CI on [10, 11]

In our study, two patients showed VEMPs before cochlear implantation and also showed VEMPs after cochlear implantation with the cochlear implant switched on. This suggests that in these cases the sensory cells of both saccule and inferior vestibular neurons may be present. One patient showed no VEMPs before cochlear implantation, but showed VEMPs with the cochlear implantation on. This suggests that in this case the sensory cells of saccule may be absent, but the inferior vestibular neurons may by present.

Our results show that among the patients with inner ear malformations and CND, there were two patients with sensory cells of saccule and inferior vestibular neurons and at least five patients with inferior vestibular neurons only, but no patients without sensory cells and vestibular neurons, as determined on the basis of VEMPs (Table 11.1). It was revealed that sensory cells of sacculus or inferior vestibular neurons or both are present in cochlear implant patients with inner ear malformations and CND, particularly common cavity deformity, using VEMPs [15].

References

1. Sheykholeslami K, Megerian CA, Arnold JE, Kaga K. Vestibular-evoked myogenic potentials in infancy and early childhood. Laryngoscope. 2005;115:1440–4. doi:10.1097/01. mlg.0000167976.58724.22.
2. Kaga K. Development of balance and motor function achieved by central vestibular compensation. Adv Neurol Sci. 2005;49:216–28.
3. Colebatch JG, Halmagyi GM, Skuse NF. Myogenic potentials generated by a click-evoked vestibulocollic reflex. J Neurol Neurosurg Psychiatry. 1994;57:190–7. doi:10.1136/jnnp.57.2.190.
4. Sheykholeslami K, Kaga. The otolithic organ as a receptor of vestibular hearing revealed by vestibular-evoked myogenic potentials in patients with inner ear anomalies. Hear Res. 2002;165:62–7. doi:10.1016/S0378-5955(02)00278-2.
5. Sheykholeslami K, Habiby Kermany M, Kaga K. Frequency sensitivity range of the saccule to bone-conducted stimuli measured by vestibular evoked myogenic potentials. Hear Res. 2001;160:58–62. doi:10.1016/S0378-5995(01)00333-1.
6. Watson SRD, Colebatch JG. Vestibulocollic reflexes evoked by short-duration galvanic stimulation in man. J Physiol. 1998;513:587–97. doi:10.1111/j.1469-7793.1998.587bb.x.
7. Sheykholeslami K, Habiby Kermany M, Kaga K. Bone-conducted vestibular evoked myogenic potentials in patients with congenital atresia of the external auditory canal. Int J Pediatr Otorhinolaryngol. 2001;57:25–9. doi:10.1016/S0165-5876(00)00430-4.
8. Shinjo Y, Jin Y, Kaga K. Assessment of vestibular function of infants and children with congenital and acquired deafness using the ice-water caloric test, rotation chair test and vestibular-evoked myogenic potential recording. Acta Otolaryngol (Stockh). 2007;127:736–47. doi:10.1080/00016480601002039.
9. Tien HC, Linthicum Jr FH. Histopathologic changes in the vestibular after cochlear implantation. Otolaryngol Head Neck Surg. 2002;127:260–4. doi:10.1067/mhn.2002.128555.
10. Jin Y, Nakamura M, Shinjo Y, Kaga K. Vestibular-evoked myogenic potentials in cochlear implant children. Acta Otolaryngol (Stockh). 2006;126:164–9. doi:10.1080/00016480500312562.
11. Jin Y, Shinjo Y, Akamatsu Y, Ogata E, Nakamura M, Yamasoba T, et al. Vestibular evoked myogenic potentials evoked by multichannel cochlear implant-influence of C levels. Acta Otolaryngol (Stockh). 2008;128:284–90. doi:10.1080/00016480701558872.
12. Jacklar RK, Luxford WM, House WF. Congenital malformations of the inner ear: a classification based on embryogenesis. Laryngoscope. 1987;97:2–14. doi:10.1002/lary.5540971301.
13. Kaga K, Suzuki JI, Roger RM, Tanaka Y. Influence of labyrinthine hypoactivity on gross motor development of infants. Ann N Y Acad Sci. 1981;374:412–20. doi:10.1111/j.1749-6632.1981.tb30887.x.
14. Anson BJ, Donaldson JA. Surgical anatomy of the temporal bone. New York: Raven; 1992.
15. Kaga K. Vertigo and balance disorders in children. Tokyo: Springer; 2014. doi:10.1007/978-4-431-54761-7.

Chapter 12
Speech and Hearing after Cochlear Implantation in Children with Inner Ear Malformation and Cochlear Nerve Deficiency

Yasushi Naito, Saburo Moroto, Hiroshi Yamazaki, and Ippei Kishimoto

Abstract Despite wide possibilities of morphological deformities, our series have shown prevalence of several malformation types, IP-II (incomplete partition type II) being most frequent followed by IP-I (incomplete partition type I) and CC (common cavity). The speech perception and production outcomes after cochlear implantation were best in IP-II, which were comparable to those in controls without malformation, followed by IP-I and CC. It is important to note, however, that significant improvement in speech perception was observed even in CC anomaly, which is the severest malformation included in the present study. The number of functioning electrodes was less than default in some ears with CC and IP-I deformities, and adjustments of the current level and pulse width were necessary in some electrodes in these groups. The electrophysiological and audiometric data in CC deformity indicated that auditory neuronal elements are mainly distributed in the anteroinferior part of the cavity. Both the relative diameter of the vestibulocochlear nerve and the presence or absence of reproducible electrically evoked brainstem responses were significantly associated with cochlear implant outcomes in patients with cochlear nerve deficiency.

Keywords Common cavity • Incomplete partition • Map • Speech perception • Electrode • Spiral ganglion neurons • Cochlear nerve deficiency • EABR

Y. Naito (✉) • S. Moroto
Department of Otolaryngology, Kobe City Medical Center General Hospital,
2-2-1, Minatojima-minamimachi, Chuo-ku, Kobe 650-0047, Japan
e-mail: naito@kcho.jp

H. Yamazaki • I. Kishimoto
Department of Otolaryngology and Head and Neck Surgery, Kyoto University graduate school of medicine, Kyoto 606-8507, Japan

© Springer Science+Business Media Singapore 2017
K. Kaga (ed.), *Cochlear Implantation in Children with Inner Ear Malformation and Cochlear Nerve Deficiency*, Modern Otology and Neurotology,
DOI 10.1007/978-981-10-1400-0_12

Table 12.1 Inner ear anomalies that underwent cochlear implantation in Kobe City Medical Center General Hospital

Anomalies		Number of ears	Number of patients
Inner ear	Common cavity[a]	10	10
	IP-I	13	11
	IP-II	18	14
	EVA	9	7
	CH-III[b]	6	3
	Lateral canal hypoplasia	1	1
	unclassified[c]	3	3
Internal auditory canal	IAC stenosis	3	2
	CNC stenosis	6	6
Total		69	57

CC common cavity, *IP* incomplete partition, *EVA* enlarged vestibular aqueduct, *CH* cochlear hypoplasia, *IAC* internal auditory canal, *CNC* cochlear nerve canal
[a]Five ears were with cochlear nerve deficiency
[b]Two patients had CHARGE syndrome, three ears with IAC stenosis, one ear with CNC stenosis, and two ears with duplicate IACs
[c]Waardenburg syndrome, CHARGE syndrome, and Down syndrome with inner ear anomaly

12.1 Introduction

Morphological abnormalities of the inner ear vary widely since there are multiple sites that can be malformed: the cochlea, the vestibule, and the internal auditory canal. The anomalies encountered in clinical practice, however, are not equally distributed, but several types prevail and others are rare. The number of the ears and patients who had inner ear and/or internal auditory canal anomalies and underwent cochlear implantation (CI) in our clinic is shown in Table 12.1. The IP-II anomaly was most frequent (26 % of all ears with anomalies), followed by IP-I (19 %) and common cavity (CC) (14 %). As for the anomaly of the internal auditory canal (IAC), stenosis of cochlear nerve canal (CNC) was more frequent than IAC stenosis. Not only inner ear and IAC anomalies but also hypoplasty of the cochlear nerve (cochlear nerve deficiency or CND) influence CI outcomes. In this chapter, we report CI outcomes of patients with inner ear anomalies, focusing on CC, IP-I, IP-II, and CND, and discuss on their pathophysiologies.

12.2 Speech Perception in CC, IP-I, and IP-II

12.2.1 Introduction

Common cavity anomaly lacks separation between the cochlear and vestibular part of the inner ear. In contrast, the cochlear and vestibular regions are individually identified in the inner ear of IP-I and IP-II, but both lack bony partitions within the cochlea,

Table 12.2 The subjects included in the present investigation

	Age at surgery (months)	Concomitant CND	Electrode array	Follow-up period (months)	CI-aided threshold (dB)
CC: 7 ears	30.4 ± 6.1	2 ears	CI24M: 1 ear, CI24RE(ST): 4 ears, CI422: 2 ears	35.8 ± 9.8	41.1 ± 3.9
IP-I: 9 ears	32.5 ± 20.4	None	CI24RE(ST): 8 ears, CI24R(CA): 1 ear	35.4 ± 9.1	34.9 ± 4.1
IP-II: 11 ears	71.1 ± 55.8	None	CI24M: 2 ears, CI24R(CS): 3 ears, CI24RE(CA): 5 ears, 90 K: 1 ear	35.8 ± 9.1	30.3 ± 4.1
Controls: 22 ears	32.8 ± 18.3	None	CI24R(CS): 1 ear, CI24RE(CA): 20 ears, 90 K: 1 ear	37.7 ± 13.9	28.4 ± 1.7

Aided thresholds = (500 Hz + 1,000 Hz + 2,000 Hz + 4,000 Hz)/4, controls: GJB2 gene mutation without anomaly
CND cochlear nerve deficiency, *CI* cochlear implant, *CC* common cavity, *IP-I* incomplete partition type I, *IP-II* incomplete partition type II

partly or completely. While the osseous structure of the basal turn including the modiolus is formed in IP-II, the bony modiolus is missing in IP-I. Thus, the primary auditory neurons exist at the center of the cochlea in IP-II, while the distribution of auditory neurons of IP-I varies and is not always located at the central region in the cochlea. Since patients with common cavity and IP-I anomalies have profound deafness at birth, cochlear implantation is the only strategy for them to obtain auditory perception. In contrast, patients with IP-II anomaly often have residual hearing, primarily in low frequencies, at birth, and there are children who acquire spoken language with hearing aids. Their hearings, however, usually deteriorate with age, and cochlear implants take over the role of hearing aids. Anatomical differences among these anomalies influence postoperative hearing and spoken language development.

12.2.2   Speech Perception Test Results

We performed cochlear implantation in 69 ears of 57 pediatric patients with malformations in the inner ear and/or in the internal auditory canal. Among them, 27 patients reached the age range at which speech perception test was possible and had been followed up more than 1 year after surgery. The test results of 27 ears in these patients, 7 ears with CC, 9 with IP-I, and 11 with IP-II anomaly, were studied (Table 12.2). The results of 22 pediatric CI patients whose hearing loss had been confirmed to be due to GJB2 gene mutation and without inner ear malformation were used as controls. Children with mental retardation and pervasive developmental disorders were excluded from the current study.

The mean age at implantation in IP-II was 71.1 months, which was much higher than the other groups (Table 12.2). The delay of CI surgery in IP-II children was due to their usable residual hearings that enabled them to, at least partly, acquire speech. But they lost hearing afterward and underwent cochlear implantation.

12.2.2.1 CI-Aided Thresholds

The CI-aided thresholds in CC, IP-I, IP-II, and control group are listed in Table 12.2. The thresholds of patients were highest in CC group, followed by IP-I. The aided thresholds of IP-II group were significantly lower than those of CC and IP-I, exhibiting no significant difference between controls.

12.2.2.2 Monosyllable Perception Scores

The monosyllable perception scores in each group are shown in Fig. 12.1. The scores were lowest in CC, followed by IP-I. The scores in IP-II and the control groups were about 80–90 % and did not differ from each other. The scores in CC and IP-I groups were significantly lower than those in IP-II and control groups.

12.2.2.3 Word Perception Scores

Figure 12.2 shows the word perception scores of CC, IP-I, IP-II, and control groups. The results are similar to monosyllable perception scores. The mean score of IP-II was 93.7 %, which was very close to 95.3 % in controls. The scores for IP-I and CC were 82.2 % and 54.3 %, respectively, which were lower than those of IP-II and controls, but the difference between each group is smaller compared to monosyllable tests.

12.2.2.4 CAP Score and SIR Scale

To assess the spoken language development in daily life situations, we examined Categories of Auditory Performance (CAP) and Speech Intelligibility Rating (SIR) Scale.

Categories of Auditory Performance (CAP) is an index consisting of eight performance categories arranged in order of increasing difficulty [1]. The category 0 means no awareness of environmental sound, 1 awareness of environmental sounds, 2 response to speech sounds, 3 identification of environmental sounds, 4 discrimination of speech sounds, 5 understanding of phrases without lip reading, 6 understanding of

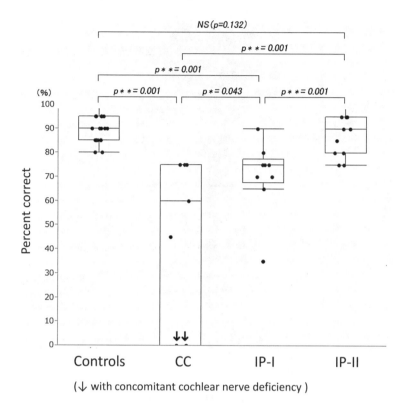

Fig. 12.1 Monosyllable perception scores

conversation without lip reading, and 7 use of the telephone. The mean CAP score in IP-II group was 6.4, which was the same as in control group, corresponding to the level of understanding conversation without lip reading, and sometimes telephone can be used. The mean scores of IP-I and CC children were 5.7 and 4.5, respectively, which were one and two levels below that of IP-II and controls (Fig. 12.3).

The Speech Intelligibility Rating (SIR) Scale is used as a framework to rank the child's spontaneous speech production into one of five hierarchic categories: (1) pre-recognizable words in spoken language, (2) connected speech is unintelligible but is developing for single words, (3) connected speech is intelligible to a listener who concentrates and lip-reads within a known context, (4) connected speech is intelligible to a listener who has little experience of a deaf person's speech (the listener does not need to concentrate unduly), and (5) connected speech is intelligible to all listeners (the child is easily understood in everyday contexts). SIR is not a performance test and was designed as a time-effective global outcome measure of speech production in real-life situations [2]. The mean SIR scores were as high as 4.8 and 4.6 in IP-II and control groups, and, again, the scores were 1 and 2 points lower in IP-I and CC groups, respectively (Fig. 12.4).

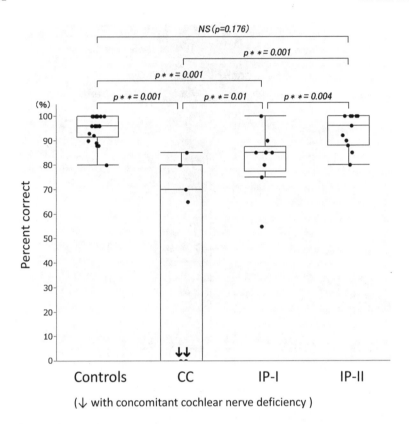

Fig. 12.2 Word perception scores

12.2.3 Mapping Characteristics in Children with an Inner Ear Anomaly

The CIs used in the current pediatric patients were all cochlear devices. In principle, electrode arrays with straight configuration (CI24M, CI24RE-ST, CI422) were selected in CC and IP-I patients, with an exception in which pre-curved electrode (CI24R-CS) was used in one IP-I patient. In contrast, pre-curved arrays (CI24R-CS, CI24RE-CA) were used more in IP-II and in control group with three exceptions in which straight-type electrode arrays (two CI24M and one CI422) were selected. The initial values of mapping parameters, pulse width, stimulation rate, and maxima (the number of electrodes for stimulation to extract sound features), are set at 25 μs, 900 Hz, and 8, respectively. The map for each patient is created by gradually raising the sound intensity from the T level (threshold level) until the charge reaches the C level (maximum comfort level) by observing the responses to the sound. If the charge amount corresponding to T level and C level is not attainable within default current range, a pulse width is widened to create a map at lower current levels. Such

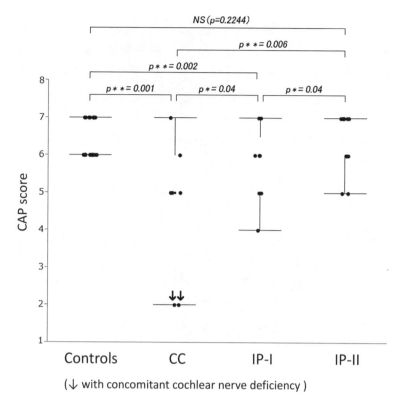

Fig. 12.3 CAP scores

adjustments are often necessary in anomalous inner ears, and there are even cases in which certain electrodes are determined to be unusable due to lack of auditory responses in spite of thorough adjustments.

12.2.3.1   Number of Usable Electrodes

The numbers of usable electrodes that elicited auditory responses ranged from 8 to 22 in CC group, 18–22 in IP-I group, and all 22 in IP-II group (Table 12.3). The numbers of usable electrodes were less in patients with smaller cavities in CC group.

12.2.3.2   The Amount of Charge Used in Electrodes

The amount of charge per phase for T levels (mean ± standard deviation) was 26.3 ± 13.4 nC for the CC group, 12.8 ± 3.3 nC for the IP-I group, 5.6 ± 1.8 nC for the IP-II group, and 4.7 ± 1.3 nC for the control group (Table 12.3). The amount of

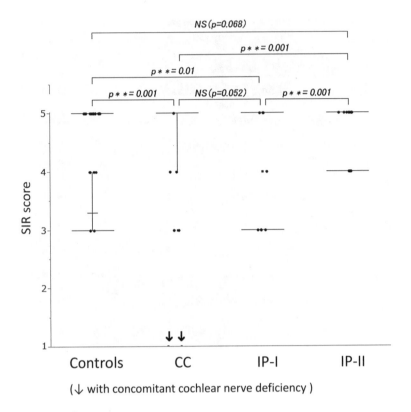

Fig. 12.4 SIR scale scores

charge used in the CC and IP-I groups was significantly greater than that of the control group ($p < 0.01$). There was no significant difference between the IP-II and control groups.

The amount of C level charge was 66.3 ± 35.1 nC for the CC group, 29.3 ± 5.3 nC for the IP-I group, and 15.4 ± 6.5 nC for the IP-II group, while it was 12.7 ± 3.4 nC for the control group (Table 12.3). Charge in CC and IP-I groups was significantly greater than that in the control group ($p < 0.01$). Again, there was no significant difference between the IP-II and control groups.

12.2.3.3 Modification of Routine Mapping Procedures

Our initial setting for pulse width was 25 μs, which was sufficient for one ear in the CC group (14.3 %), one ear in the IP-I group (11 %), and all ears in the IP-II and the control groups (Table 12.3). There was a need to set the pulse width wider than 25 μs in six ears in the CC group and eight ears in the IP-I group. Of these 14 ears, for two ears in the CC group and for six ears in the IP-I group, it was possible to ensure the appropriate amount of charge corresponding to C level by expanding the

Table 12.3 Mapping parameters

Groups	Number of functioning electrodes	Amount of charge per phase for T and C levels (nC)[a] (mean ± SD)		Pulse width and facial stimulation below C level		
		T level	C level	Pulse width =25 μs	Pulse width >25 μs without facial nerve stimulation	Facial stimulation below C level
CC (7 ears)	8 (1 ear)	26.3 ± 13.4[b]	66.3 ± 35.1[b]	1 ear (14.3 %)	2 ears (28.6 %)	4 ears (57.1)%
	17 (2 ears)					
	22 (4 ears)					
IP-I (9 ears)	18 (1 ear)	12.8 ± 3.3[b]	29.3 ± 5.3[b]	1 ear (11 %)	6 ears (67 %)	2 ears (22 %)
	22 (8 ears)					
IP-II (11 ears)	22 (all 11 ears)	5.6 ± 1.8	15.4 ± 6.5	11 ears (100 %)	None	None
Controls (22 ears)	22 (all 22 ears)	4.7 ± 1.3	12.7 ± 3.4	22 ears (100 %)	None	None

CC common cavity, *IP-I* incomplete partition type I, *IP-II* incomplete partition type II
[a]Amount of charge in nanocoulomb (nC) = amount of current (μ A) × pulse width (μs) × 1000
[b]$P < 0.01$ larger than controls (Kruskal-Wallis, Mann-Whitney U test, Bonferroni correction)

pulse width from 37 to 88 μs and without encountering facial nerve stimulation. Nevertheless, for four ears in the CC group and two ears in the IP-I group (Table 12.3), increasing the current level stimulated the facial nerve, and securing a charge amount corresponding to the C level was challenging. As a result of re-adjusting the map through further expansion of pulse width, for five out of the six ears, we were able to reach C level before encountering facial nerve stimulation. Nevertheless, for the one remaining ear, it was not possible to suppress the facial nerve stimulation, and maximum stimulation remained at a lower value than the charge amount corresponding to the C level.

12.3 Discussion on Speech Perception and Map Parameters

The results of cochlear implantation in patients with inner ear malformations have been reported by many authors. Despite wide possibilities of morphological deformities, our series have shown prevalence of several malformation types, IP-II being most frequent followed by IP-I and CC, which is similar to previous results including the one by Sennaroglu et al. [3]. These findings indicate general patterns for inner ear malformation occurrence and the importance of detailed analysis on CI outcomes in CC, IP-I, and IP-II.

It is important to check whether patients with mental retardation or developmental disorder are included in the study or not when interpreting the CI outcomes of patients with inner ear malformations. In overall, children suffering from developmental disorder [4] or mental retardation [4, 5] do not progress as well as the non-delayed children after cochlear implantation. In the current study, we excluded patients with developmental disorders and those with mental retardation. Thus, our results may reflect the difference in inner ear morphology and spiral ganglion cells between malformation and normal anatomy cases.

On speech perception and production outcomes, the results in IP-II were comparable to those in controls and significantly better than those observed in CC and IP-I, which are in line with the findings in previous studies [6–8]. Although osseous modiolus and interscalar septa of cochlear upper turns are missing in IP-II anomaly, neurosensory elements and SG cells exist not only in the basal turn but in the upper region in approximately the same location as in the cochlea without anomaly [9], which may be the reason for IP-II's good CI outcomes. We may not have to expect significant disadvantage in CI-mediated speech perception in patients with IP-II anomaly when considering their indication for CI.

Although speech perception scores of CC patients using CI were lower than those in IP-II and control groups, it is important to note that significant improvement in speech perception was observed even in CC anomaly, which is the severest malformation included in the present study. Similar positive effects of CI on spoken language development in CC patients have been reported [7, 8].

The number of functioning electrodes was less than default in three ears in CC and one ear in IP-I groups, but all electrodes could be activated in all ears in IP-II and in control groups. Vera et al. [10] also reported that the number of functioning electrodes was significantly less in patients with malformed inner ear compared to those in patients without malformation. Significant differences were observed between the major and minor malformation groups in their study. As for mapping parameters, we found that the amount of charge per phase for T and C levels was significantly higher in CC and IP-I groups, which is also the same tendency observed in the previous investigation [10]. In most patients in CC and IP-I groups in the present study, pulse width had to be adjusted wider than the default value of 25 µs, suggesting that more charge was necessary to activate sufficient number of SG neurons and bring about sound sensation.

In the present study, four (60 %) of the seven CC patients and two (22 %) of the nine IP-I patients experienced CI-mediated facial nerve stimulation (FNS), which is consistent with the previous study reporting the high frequency of FNS among patients with inner ear malformations who had implants [11–13]. In cases with a severe inner ear malformation, high current level and/or increased pulse width are often required to achieve good auditory performance [13, 14], suggesting a necessity to adjust the current level to an appropriate value that is high enough to provide sufficient auditory input but lower than the threshold for FNS. The stimulus amplitude cannot be increased higher if it reaches the level of facial nerve stimulation, which practically limits the dynamic range of the CI map.

Lack of tonotopy in the cochlea and smaller number of SG neurons in inner ears with malformations [15–17] may underlie their relatively lower CI outcomes. It has been reported that at least 10,000 SG neurons may be necessary for speech discrimination by CI [18]. However, there is also a report discussing that benefit from CI can be obtained in patients with as few as 3,300 SG cells [19]. Kahn et al. [20] reported that significant correlation between psychophysical measures and SG neuron counts was found in only two of the five subjects they examined. Auditory perception by CI with fewer SG cells may be achieved by higher neural synchrony of SG cells activated by direct electrical stimulation. Possible redundancy in cochlear innervation [6] and plastic reorganization of cortical language networks [21] may also contribute to successful perception and production of speech through CI. The shape and placement of the electrode array in the inner ear cavity, especially in CC deformity, influence the outcomes of CI, which will be discussed in the following section.

12.4 Distribution of Auditory Neurons in Common Cavity Anomaly

12.4.1 Introduction

Effective stimulation of SG neurons by CI electrodes is necessary for better CI outcome, but the spatial distribution of SG cells and auditory nerve fibers is unclear in CC deformity because of no differentiation between the cochlea and vestibule in addition to the lack of a modiolus. Electrically evoked auditory brainstem responses (EABRs) using CI-mediated stimulus can be used for the objective evaluation of auditory neuronal responses in the brainstem [6, 14, 22]. In this section, we show the results of our previous EABR investigation [23] on the spatial distribution of auditory neurons in CC deformity.

12.4.2 CI-Mediated EABR Findings in CC Patients

We retrospectively examined five patients with CC deformity with congenital profound sensorineural hearing loss who underwent cochlear implantation at our hospital from 2005 to 2013. Mean age at implantation was 27.4 months, and the mean follow-up period was 26.0 months. Nucleus device with 22 active electrodes (Ch1–Ch22), including CI24RST, CI24REST, or CI422, was implanted in all cases. Intraoperative EABR testing was performed with Nucleus Custom Sound EP software using MP 1 + 2 mode. The EABR was recorded with a filter setting of 20 Hz to 3 kHz on the opposite side to minimize artifacts of the implanted device.

In Case 1 (Fig. 12.5), the radiograph obtained during the initial cochlear implantation demonstrated that most of the electrodes were located within the CC deformity, but the CI-aided performance was still poor even after 1 year of use of CI. EABR elicited a reproducible evoked wave V (eV) only at 2 of 11 tested electrodes. Thus,

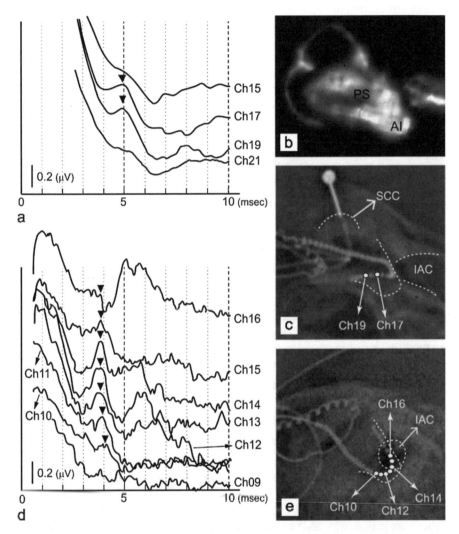

Fig. 12.5 Results of EABR testing in Case 1 before and after the reimplantation. (**a**) EABR testing after the initial implantation with the showing eVs in Ch17 and Ch19 among the 11 tested electrodes. The latency of these eVs is approximately 5 ms (*arrowheads*). (**b**) A maximum intensity projection of the T2-weighted magnetic resonance image of the CC deformity on the implanted side. The anteroinferior part of the CC deformity (AI) is smaller than the posterosuperior part (PS). (**c**) Radiograph of the initial implantation. (**d**) EABR testing after the reimplantation showing a distinct eV in 7 of 22 electrodes. The latency of these eVs ranges from 3.8 to 4.1 ms (*arrowheads*). (**e**) Radiograph after the reimplantation demonstrating that electrodes with a positive eV (*circles*) are located in the anteroinferior part of the CC deformity (*dotted line*) (Cited from Ref. [23] with permission)

we performed reimplantation surgery with wider labyrinthotomy, resulting in successful placement of the electrode array in the anteroinferior region of the inner ear cavity, obtaining appropriate eV at seven electrodes. In the other four patients, postoperative CT images showed the optimal position of the electrode array, requiring no revision surgery. Although the size and shape of each CC deformity differed among the cases (Fig. 12.6a–d), electrodes inserted in the anteroinferior cavity successfully elicited eVs in all four cases, similarly to Case 1 (Fig. 12.6e–h).

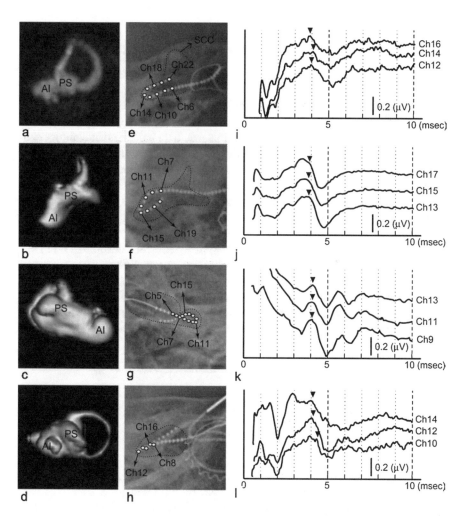

Fig. 12.6 Results of EABR testing in Cases 2–5. (**a–d**) Maximum intensity projection of T2-weighted magnetic resonance images of the CC deformity on the implanted side. *AI* and *PS* indicate the anteroinferior and posterosuperior parts of the CC. (**e–h**) Electrodes with a positive eV (*circles*) are located in the anteroinferior part of the CC. (**i–l**) EABRs for three representative electrodes. The latency of these eVs is approximately 4 ms in all cases (*arrowheads*) (Cited from Ref. [23] with permission)

Before implantation, no patient could detect sounds, that is, their preoperative CAP score was zero, but auditory perception improved after activation of the CI in all patients. The postoperative CAP score reached to 6 in Cases 1 and 2 who had used their CI for more than 2 years, and their speech discrimination scores of closed-set infant words were 76 % and 80 %, respectively. The other three patients, Cases 3, 4, and 5, who had used their CI for less than 2 years, showed CAP scores of 4, 3, and 3, respectively, and Case 3 showed 40 % of the infant word discrimination score.

12.4.3   Discussion on CI-Mediated EABR in Common Cavity Anomaly

The present results demonstrated that reproducible eVs were elicited by activating electrodes that were located at the anteroinferior part of the CC deformity in all patients. The electrophysiological and audiometric data indicate that auditory neuronal elements are mainly distributed in the anteroinferior part of the CC deformity. In the normal development of an inner ear, the ventral portion of the otic vesicle elongates in the ventral direction, initiating cochlear development [24]; therefore, the anteroinferior part of CC deformity might be programmed to differentiate to a cochlea. These findings support our conclusion regarding the anteroinferior distribution of auditory neuronal tissue in CC deformity.

Case 1 who showed eV only at 7 (31.8 %) of 22 electrodes exhibited 6 in CAP score and 76 % in the infant word discrimination test at 4 years after the initial implantation, which are similar to those observed in the 2-year postoperative Case 2 who showed eV at almost all electrodes (81.8 %). These data suggest that even if the only limited number of electrodes shows eV in EABR testing, the patient might achieve sufficient CI-aided auditory performance after long-term use of the CI with an appropriate program.

12.5   Cochlear Nerve Deficiency

12.5.1   Introduction

Hypoplasia and aplasia of the cochlear branch of the vestibulocochlear nerve, called cochlear nerve deficiency (CND), are defined by an absent or a small cochlear branch of the vestibulocochlear nerve (cochlear nerve) on MRI [25–27]. Several studies have reported that congenitally deaf children with CND show significantly poorer auditory performance using CI than children without CND [26, 28]. However, many patients with CND understood some words in a closed-set word discrimination test using CI [26, 28]. Previous studies investigating CI children with CND demonstrated that the CI outcomes were correlated to the type of malformation on CT and MRI and the result of intracochlear EABR [26, 28]. In this section, we show the results of our previous collaborative research by the University of Melbourne and Kobe City Medical Center General Hospital [29], aiming to establish a strategy of preoperative and intraoperative objective examinations to discriminate CND patients with poor CI outcomes from those with satisfactory CI outcomes.

12.5.2 Patients, Methods, and Results

A retrospective examination of 19 congenital deaf children with CND who underwent cochlear implantation at Kobe City Medical Center General Hospital or Melbourne Cochlear Implant Clinic from 2003 to 2013 was conducted. The mean age at implantation was 26.7 ± 11.5 months, and the median follow-up period was 34 months. Nucleus devices were implanted. Simultaneous and sequential bilateral cochlear implantations were performed in one and four children, respectively.

Narrow internal auditory canal (NIAC) was defined by the width of midpoint of the IAC being narrower than 2 mm [6]. Hypoplasia of bony cochlear nerve canal (HBCNC) was defined by less than 1.4 mm in the diameter of the bony cochlear nerve canal as well as a normal width of the IAC on CT images [25]. NIAC was identified on the implanted side of six patients, HBCNC in six patients, cochlear aplasia (CA) in one patient, CC in five patients, and CH-III in two patients. MRI was acquired using a 1.5-T or 3.0-T system, which failed to visualize a definitive bundle of a cochlear nerve at the fundus of the IAC in all patients, on the basis of which CND was diagnosed. For each case, the relative diameter of the vestibulocochlear nerve compared to the facial nerve was evaluated at the cerebellopontine angle (CPA). The vestibulocochlear nerve was smaller than the facial nerve at the CPA in seven children, whereas it was equal to or larger than the facial nerve in the remaining 12 (Fig. 12.7). Intracochlear EABR testing was performed in the operation room using Nucleus Custom Sound EP software, of which details are described in our previous report [23].

Auditory performance with the CI was evaluated using CAP scores [1]. Preoperative and postoperative CAP scores in this population with CND were 0.2 ± 0.4 and 3.0 ± 2.1, respectively, and significant improvement in the auditory performance was observed after cochlear implantation. Children with relatively thin vestibulocochlear nerves "CN7 > CN8" had significantly poorer performance: postoperative CAP scores 1.1 ± 1.5, compared to those with more normal sized nerves "CN7 <= CN8," CAP score 4.1 ± 1.5 (Fig. 12.8a). With respect to the EABR testing, the postoperative CAP score was 4.3 ± 1.2 in those with "positive eV," which is significantly higher than 1.8 ± 1.9 in those with "negative eV" (Fig. 12.8b).

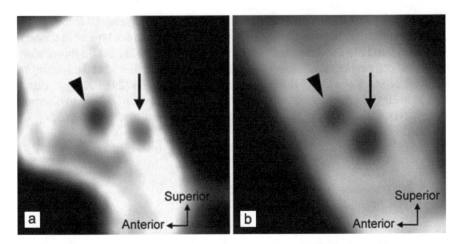

Fig. 12.7 Evaluation of relative diameter of the vestibulocochlear nerve compared to the facial nerve at CPA using MRI. MRI shows the vestibulocochlear nerve (*arrows*) and the facial nerve (*arrowheads*) at the CPA. (**a**) "CN7 > CN8," (**b**) "CN7 <= CN8" (Cited from Ref. [29] with permission)

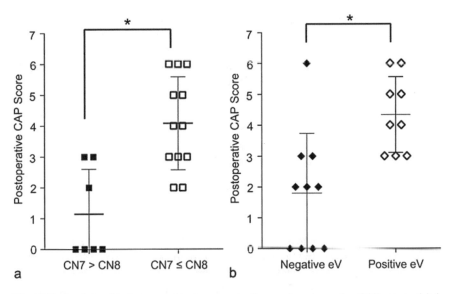

Fig. 12.8 A relationship between objective examinations and postoperative CAP scores. (**a**) A relationship between the MRI findings and postoperative CAP scores. (**b**) A relationship between the EABR results and postoperative CAP scores (Cited from Ref. [29] with permission)

Although the results of MRI and EABR testing were significantly associated with postoperative CI outcomes, each examination failed to clearly discriminate patients with poor CI outcomes from those with satisfactory CI outcomes. Combination of the results of MRI and EABR testing allowed better discrimination between children with limited or no benefit from a CI and those with moderate or good CI-aided auditory performance. All of the six patients who were categorized into both "CN7 > CN8" and "negative eV" exhibited less than or equal to 3 in the postoperative CAP scores, and four of them (66.7 %) showed no response to sound (CAP score of 0) even after 2 years of CI use. On the contrary, all of the eight children who showed "CN7 <= CN8" on MRI and "positive eV" on EABR testing reached greater than or equal to 3 in the CAP scores within 2 years after implantation, and six of them (75.0 %) discriminated at least some speech sounds without visual support (CAP score of 4).

12.5.3   Discussion on CI in Cochlear Nerve Deficiency

In this investigation, we found that both the relative diameter of the vestibulocochlear nerve in the CPA as seen on the preoperative MRI and the presence or absence of reproducible eVs with typical latency in the intraoperative EABR testing were significantly associated with postoperative auditory performance with CI. It was also demonstrated that the combination of MRI and EABR testing achieved more precise discrimination immediately after cochlear implantation between patients with no or limited benefit from CI and those with moderate to good CI outcomes than independent use of either.

CND is thought to diminish development of auditory perception with CI because of a small number of SG neurons [30]. A previous histological study showed that the count of the SG neurons was predicted by the maximum diameter of the main trunk of the vestibulocochlear nerve [31]. Theoretically, the counts of SG neurons relate to the size of the cochlear nerve more strongly than the main trunk of the vestibulocochlear nerve; however, accurate measurement of the diameter of the cochlear nerve is often difficult. Therefore, evaluation of the vestibulocochlear nerve at the CPA is reasonable to prevent underestimation in specific types of malformations.

Regarding the other groups, "CN7 > CN8/positive eV" and "CN7 <=CN8/negative eV," interpretation is not straightforward because the results of MRI and the EABR testing are contradictory. In the patient categorized in "CN7 > CN8/positive eV," the detection of eV suggests the auditory brainstem was activated by CI, but the number of SGNs was not enough to discriminate speech sounds. Among the four subjects with "CN7 <=CN8/negative eV," three children showed 2 or 3 in the postoperative CAP score, suggesting hypoplasia of the cochlear nerve component.

The current data may be informative to decide the treatment strategy in congenitally deaf children with CND.

References

1. Archbold S, Lutman ME, Marshall DH. Categories of auditory performance. Ann Otol Rhinol Laryngol Suppl. 1995;166:312–4.
2. Allen C, Nikolopoulos TP, Dyar D, O'Donoghue GM. Reliability of a rating scale for measuring speech intelligibility after pediatric cochlear implantation. Otol Neurotol. 2001;22:631–3.
3. Sennaroglu L, Sarac S, Ergin T. Surgical results of cochlear implantation in malformed cochlea. Otol Neurotol. 2006;27:615–23.
4. Yamazaki H, Yamamoto R, Moroto S, Yamazaki T, Fujiwara K, Nakai M, Ito J, Naito Y. Cochlear implantation in children with congenital cytomegalovirus infection accompanied by psycho-neurological disorders. Acta Otolaryngol. 2012;132:420–7.
5. Rachovitsas D, Psillas G, Chatzigiannakidou V, Triaridis S, Constantinidis J, Vital V. Speech perception and production in children with inner ear malformations after cochlear implantation. Int J Pediatr Otorhinolaryngol. 2012;76:1370–4.
6. Papsin BC. Cochlear implantation in children with anomalous cochleovestibular anatomy. Laryngoscope. 2005;115(1 Pt 2 Suppl 106):1–26.
7. Xia J, Wang W, Zhang D. Cochlear implantation in 21 patients with common cavity malformation. Acta Otolaryngol. 2015;135:459–65.
8. Pakdaman MN, Herrmann BS, Curtin HD, Van Beek-King J, Lee DJ. Cochlear implantation in children with anomalous cochleovestibular anatomy: a systematic review. Otolaryngol Head Neck Surg. 2012;146:180–90.
9. Leung KJ, Quesnel AM, Juliano AF, Curtin HD. Correlation of CT, MR, and histopathology in incomplete partition-II cochlear anomaly. Otol Neurotol. 2016;37:434–7.
10. Palomeque Vera JM, Gómez-Hervás J, Fernández-Prada M, Alba-Saida GN, González Ramírez AR, Sainz Quevedo M. Effectiveness of cochlear implant in inner ear bone malformations with anterior labyrinth involvement. Int J Pediatr Otorhinolaryngol. 2015;79:369–73.
11. Cushing SL, Papsin BC, Gordon KA. Incidence and characteristics of facial nerve stimulation in children with cochlear implants. Laryngoscope. 2006;116:1787–91.
12. Ahn JII, Oh SH, Chung JW, Lee KS. Facial nerve stimulation after cochlear implantation according to types of nucleus 24-channel electrode arrays. Acta Otolaryngol. 2009;129:588–91.
13. Buchman CA, Copeland BJ, Yu KK, Brown CJ, Carrasco VN, Pillsbury 3rd HC. Cochlear implantation in children with congenital inner ear malformations. Laryngoscope. 2004;114:309–16.
14. Cinar BC, Atas A, Sennaroglu G, Sennaroglu L. Evaluation of objective test techniques in cochlear implant users with inner ear malformations. Otol Neurotol. 2011;32:1065–74.
15. Sainz M, Fernández E, García-Valdecasas J, Aviñoa A. Neural distribution of hearing structures in inner ear malformations and the need of further cochlear implant stimulation strategies. Cochlear Implants Int. 2010;11 Suppl 1:204–6.
16. Monsell EM, Jackler RK, Motta G, Linthicum Jr FH. Congenital malformations of the inner ear: histologic findings in five temporal bones. Laryngoscope. 1987;97(3 Pt 2 Suppl 40):18–24.
17. Miura M, Sando I, Hirsch BE, Orita Y. Analysis of spiral ganglion cell populations in children with normal and pathological ears. Ann Otol Rhinol Laryngol. 2002;111(12 Pt 1):1059–65.
18. Otte J, Schuknecht HF, Kerr AG. Ganglion cell populations in normal and pathological human cochleae. Implications for cochlear implantation. Laryngoscope. 1978;88:1231–46.
19. Linthicum Jr FH, Fayad J, Otto SR, Galey FR, House WF. Cochlear implant histopathology. Am J Otol. 1991;12:245–311.
20. Khan AM, Whiten DM, Nadol Jr JB, Eddington DK. Histopathology of human cochlear implants: correlation of psychophysical and anatomical measures. Hear Res. 2005;205:83–93.
21. Naito Y, Tateya I, Fujiki N, Hirano S, Ishizu K, Nagahama Y, Fukuyama H, Kojima H. Increased cortical activation during hearing of speech in cochlear implant users. Hear Res. 2000;143:139–46.

22. Gordon KA, Papsin BC, Harrison RV. Activity-dependent developmental plasticity of the auditory brain stem in children who use cochlear implants. Ear Hear. 2003;24:485–500.
23. Yamazaki H, Naito Y, Fujiwara K, Moroto S, Yamamoto R, Yamazaki T, Sasaki I. Electrically evoked auditory brainstem response-based evaluation of the spatial distribution of auditory neuronal tissue in common cavity deformities. Otol Neurotol. 2014;35:1394–402.
24. Kelley MW. Development of the inner ear. New York: Springer; 2005. xii, 240 p.
25. Adunka OF, Jewells V, Buchman CA. Value of computed tomography in the evaluation of children with cochlear nerve deficiency. Otol Neurotol. 2007;28:597–604.
26. Buchman CA, Teagle HF, Roush PA, Park LR, Hatch D, Woodard J, Zdanski C, Adunka OF. Cochlear implantation in children with labyrinthine anomalies and cochlear nerve deficiency: implications for auditory brainstem implantation. Laryngoscope. 2011;121:1979–88.
27. Kutz Jr JW, Lee KH, Isaacson B, Booth TN, Sweeney MH, Roland PS. Cochlear implantation in children with cochlear nerve absence or deficiency. Otol Neurotol. 2011;32:956–61.
28. Valero J, Blaser S, Papsin BC, James AL, Gordon KA. Electrophysiologic and behavioral outcomes of cochlear implantation in children with auditory nerve hypoplasia. Ear Hear. 2012;33:3–18.
29. Yamazaki H, Leigh J, Briggs R, Naito Y. Usefulness of MRI and EABR testing for predicting CI outcomes immediately after cochlear implantation in cases with cochlear nerve deficiency. Otol Neurotol. 2015;36:977–84.
30. Nelson EG, Hinojosa R. Aplasia of the cochlear nerve: a temporal bone study. Otol Neurotol. 2001;22:790–5.
31. Nadol Jr JB, Xu WZ. Diameter of the cochlear nerve in deaf humans: implications for cochlear implantation. Ann Otol Rhinol Laryngol. 1992;101:988–93.

Index

© Springer Science+Business Media Singapore 2017
K. Kaga (ed.), *Cochlear Implantation in Children with Inner Ear Malformation
and Cochlear Nerve Deficiency*, Modern Otology and Neurotology,
DOI 10.1007/978-981-10-1400-0

Printed in the United States
By Bookmasters